Books are to be returned on or before
the last date below.

D1580945

Organ and Tissue Don.
An Evidence Base for Practice

/Wi.

LIVERPOOL JMU LIBRARY

3 1111 01207 2219

Organ and Tissue Donation: An Evidence Base for Practice

Edited by Magi Sque and Sheila Payne

 Open University Press
Maidenhead ● New York

Open University Press
McGraw-Hill Education
McGraw-Hill House
Shoppenhangers Road
Maidenhead
Berkshire
England
SL6 2QL

email: enquiries@openup.co.uk
world wide web: www.openup.co.uk

and Two Penn Plaza, New York, NY 10121–2289, USA

First published 2007

Copyright © Authors and Contributors 2007

All rights reserved. Except for the quotation of short passages for the purposes of
criticism and review, no part of this publication may be reproduced, stored in a
retrieval system, or transmitted, in any form, or by any means, electronic,
mechanical, photocopying, recording or otherwise, without the prior permission
of the publisher or a licence from the Copyright Licensing Agency Limited. Details
of such licences (for reprographic reproduction) may be obtained from the
Copyright Licensing Agency Ltd of 6–10 Kirby Street, London, EC1N 8TS.

A catalogue record of this book is available from the British Library

ISBN 10: 0335 216 927 (pb) 0335 216 935 (hb)
ISBN 13: 9780 335 216 925 (pb) 9780 335 216 932 (hb)

Library of Congress Cataloguing-in-Publication Data
CIP data applied for

Typeset by YHT Ltd, London
Printed in Poland by OZ Graf S.A. www.polskabook.pl

The McGraw·Hill Companies

Contents

To
Michael Sque
Verity, Sebastian, Kyle, Thomas
and
Ken Payne

List of contributors

Alison K. Crombie is a visiting Reader at South Bank University and Associate Director of Education at Barking, Havering and Redbridge Trust. Her Ph.D. from Brunel University focused on the social and cultural issues of living donation from the perspective of biomedical colleagues and individual donors and recipients. Alison has published on several related aspects of donation and transplantation.

Patricia M. Franklin is the Senior Clinical Nurse Specialist and Psychologist in Transplantation at the Oxford Transplant Centre. She currently leads the transplant specialist nursing team responsible for assessing, coordinating and evaluating the live donor programme. She has recently undergone training as an Independent Assessor for living donations with the new Human Tissue Authority.

Delyth Hughes is an experienced palliative care nurse currently working as a ward manager at St Raphael's Hospice. Her research interests concern organ and tissue donation within the palliative care setting. Her postgraduate research, M.Sc. in Advanced Clinical Practice, explored the knowledge and attitudes of palliative care patients towards organ and tissue donation.

Bridie Kent, Ph.D., is the Director of Clinical Nursing Research at the University of Auckland, New Zealand. She is a registered nurse and experienced educator. Her research focuses on end-of-life issues, especially decisions relating to organ and tissue donation and evidence-based practice. Her work on professionals' attitudes to tissue donation is recognized internationally.

Tracy Long is a Senior Research Fellow at University of Southampton. A chartered health psychologist she worked as transplant psychologist, at the world-renowned Harefield Hospital. Her Ph.D. is exploring the development of the diagnosis of death, based on neurological criteria, and how brainstem death is perceived, understood and synthesized by family members approached about organ donation.

Jill Macleod Clark, Ph.D., DBE, is Professor of Nursing and Head of the School of Nursing and Midwifery at the University of Southampton, and Deputy Dean of the Faculty of Medicine, Health and Life Sciences. Dame Jill has an extensive research portfolio in health promotion. She is involved nationally and internationally in professional nursing activities and is a member of the NHS Workforce Development Board.

Parul Mistry is a physician in internal medicine. She is Senior Medical Director at Executive Health Resources in Philadelphia, an organization that assists in improving hospitals and health systems. Parul holds a masters degree in bioethics from Case Western Reserve University. Her areas of interest include advance directives and issues involving end of life care.

Mary Murray, Ph.D., is a sociologist at Massey University in New Zealand. She has researched and published in the areas of historical sociology and feminist theory. Mary's research and teaching interests now lie in the areas of the sociology of death and dying, emotions, social and feminist theory and the relationship between humans and other animals. She has published in these areas including a book *The Law of the Father?* (1995).

Sheila Payne holds the Help the Hospices Chair in Hospice Studies at Lancaster University. She is a health psychologist with a background in nursing. Her research agenda focuses on two issues: palliative and end of life care for older people, and bereavement. She has been involved in developing a number of British national research organizations in palliative care and bereavement.

Ruth Richardson, D.Phil., F.R.Hist.S. has published widely on the history of medicine and lectured to academic and medical audiences worldwide. Her *Builder Illustrations Index 1843–1883* (co-authored with Robert Thorne) was awarded the Wheatley Gold Medal. Her most recent works are a new historical introduction to the latest edition of *Gray's Anatomy* (2005), and *Vintage Papers from The Lancet* (2006).

Magi Sque is a Senior Lecturer at the School of Nursing and Midwifery at the University of Southampton. She studied nursing at Guy's Hospital, London, and specialized in oncological nursing. Supported by a British Department of Health Nursing Research Studentship she completed a Ph.D. in 1996. Her research explores issues that concern bereavement, organ donation, retention and transplantation.

Joanne Wells is Nurse Consultant in Palliative Care between The Princess Alice Hospice, Esher and Kingston Hospital NHS Trust. She holds an M.Sc. in Advanced Clinical Practice and is currently engaged in doctoral research at the University of Southampton exploring corneal donation within the hospice setting.

Introduction

This book provides an evidence base for the psychological and social issues that concern families, health professionals and others involved with organ and tissue donation. In most countries worldwide human transplant technology depends on the unconditional donation of organs from the deceased, usually following a sudden and traumatic death. Legislation in some countries (e.g. Human Tissue Act 2004; Dodd-McCue *et al.* 2006) now gives precedence to the wishes of the deceased, expressed while they were alive. Therefore, families have no right to veto these wishes. However, relatives of potential deceased donors remain a critical link in maintaining organ supply, as organ donation is normally discussed with them and their support for, agreement or lack of an objection sought, before donation takes place. Therefore, at a time of often sudden and unexpected loss, relatives are asked to make or support decisions about organ and tissue donation. Little is known about how these choices are made and what the implications are for the bereaved.

Research has shown that this donation event is couched in a particular psychological and social milieu that transcends and challenges traditional understandings of death, bereavement, gift-giving, decision-making and continuation of life. This book draws together for the first time evidence which informs our understanding of work in the area of donation. The outstanding feature of the book is its strong evidence base of original research, with theoretical perspectives about the social and psychological issues that underpin organ donation.

Who is the book for?

This book is internationally applicable, especially in countries with well resourced and developed health care systems and where organ and tissue donation takes place using similar practices. It will interest a range of individuals concerned with the psychological and social issues that affect this bereaved population. The book is relevant to transplant coordinators and qualified clinical practitioners working in intensive care, accident and emergency, operating theatres, palliative care services, tissue donation services and bereavement counselling services.

It is a useful reference book for services dedicated to the national organization of donation and transplantation, hospital bereavement services, voluntary bereavement organizations, organ and tissue donation peer support groups, hospital and community chaplains, funeral directors and coroners.

The book also contributes to the end of life, palliative and bereavement care literature and is therefore recommended as a core text for post-registration and postgraduate health practitioners undertaking specialist programmes in transplant coordination, intensive care, accident and emergency, anaesthesia, operating theatre, palliative care and bereavement counselling.

The book addresses three key questions:

1   What is the historical and social context that shapes our attitudes towards and understanding of organ and tissue donation?
2   How do the bereavement experiences of organ donor families differ from other types of bereavement?
3   How can health and social care professionals support families during their decision-making about organ or tissue donation?

The first three chapters set the context in which the research information contained in the rest of the book can be understood.

Chapter 1 describes the historical context by exploring the history of human dissection from the abortive and exploitative tooth transplants of eighteenth-century England to the modern rise of organ donation in the second half of the last century. Chapter 2 introduces three theoretical perspectives on bereavement. The purpose is to enable readers to understand how conceptual models of loss and bereavement have been influential in shaping contemporary ways to talk about grief and behave during bereavement. Drawing on data from three studies Chapter 3 examines the relative value of either the 'gift of life' or 'sacrifice' as discourses that contribute to a greater understanding of organ donor families' decision-making. Chapter 4 reports a study carried out in the UK that examined, through face-to-face interviews, relatives' experiences of organ donation. Their experience was explained as a theory of 'dissonant loss'. Chapter 5 draws on a three-year, longitudinal study to explore the factors and processes that underpinned families' organ donation decision-making. Chapter 6 focuses upon the attitudes of health professionals to tissue donation in the light of recent research findings. Chapter 7 addresses tissue donation outside of the intensive care unit, drawing particularly on examples of studies about corneal donation carried out in the palliative care setting. Chapter 8 uses two anthropological studies to provide insights into family relationships, and the selection of donors by health professionals during decision-making about living donation. Chapter 9 uses a sociological perspective to consider issues of cross-species transplantation and ponders what this means to our concept of being human.

The final chapter reviews contentious issues in organ and tissue donation and transplantation, and considers visions of the future and the potential contribution of these important health interventions.

References

Dodd-McCue, D., Cowheard, R., Iverson, A. and Myer, M. (2006) Family responses to donor designation in donation cases: a longitudinal study, *Progress in Transplantation*, 16(2): 150–4.

Human Tissue Act (2004) London: HMSO.

1 Human dissection and organ transplantation in historical context

Ruth Richardson

Introduction[1]

When a nurse or a doctor wishes to examine a wound, they take away the dressings to see how things look beneath. Historians unpack the present by looking behind it, to try to discern roots and causes. This chapter looks at transplantation in a long historical context (since the sixteenth century) which includes the funerary culture of the British Isles, the judicial use of dissection as a punishment, bodysnatching, transplantation itself, and the history of bodily donation, in an attempt to help explain modern phenomena which might otherwise seem perplexing, such as organ shortage. The geographical focus is the UK, but aspects of the story have echoes elsewhere, particularly in Europe, and in countries with a history of British colonial involvement, including Australia and North America.

Although transplantation as a successful medical therapy is comparatively recent in its development, historical parallels do exist, both for the actual transplantation of body parts and the wariness with which donation is often regarded (Youngner *et al.* 1996). In the eighteenth century bodysnatching provided a source of body parts for anatomists and early transplantation efforts. Public resistance to bodysnatching also bears similarities to modern opposition to un-consented organ removal and retention (Redfern 2001). The popular revulsion toward bodysnatching, and the importance of the 1832 Anatomy Act, which sought to provide adequate supplies of bodies for the anatomists, cannot be fully understood without examining the traditional attitudes that existed toward death and the corpse. This chapter will therefore explore traditional eighteenth-century death culture; attempts by government to provide an adequate supply of corpses for anatomists; and the outrage provoked by bodysnatching when these provisions proved inadequate. The short-lived vogue for tooth transplantation in the last quarter of the eighteenth century will be briefly examined along with the reasons for its failure, and ethical and medical critiques of the day. The chapter then examines the negative cultural impact of the 1832 Anatomy Act, and its long-term effects to within living memory. It concludes on an encouraging note concerning the history of body and organ donation, which developed apace after the establishment of the National Health Service (NHS); and the en-actment of the Human Tissue Act (2004) which, it is hoped, will help safe-guard vulnerable communities both of the living and the dead.

Traditional care of the dead

The physicality of the human corpse is undeniable, making the disposal of such perishable remains imperative. Today, preparation of the dead for dis-posal is regarded as a sanitary problem, dealt with professionally by hospitals and undertakers. Modern funerary practices and language often obscure the role of the corpse in the proceedings by euphemism, affected delicacy and outright evasion. Practices were very different when a person died in the eighteenth or early nineteenth centuries, as were the traditional ways of caring for the body. Most people died at home, but if they died elsewhere, they would be brought home if that were possible. There were very few hospitals, and those served only people in desperate surgical need who could not afford to pay a surgeon. Most people avoided hospitals if they possibly could: the idea of dying in one was spurned. Even today, when hospital care is widely available and attitudes have altered considerably, most people would still much prefer to die at home (Higginson and Sen-Gupta 2000).

Traditionally, after a death the body would remain at home for several days, while arrangements were made for burial. There were no undertakers' chapels of rest or funeral homes in those days, and in fact not many under-takers either. Only very large institutions, like hospitals and prisons, might have had what was called a 'dead house'. Public mortuaries did not exist, nor did municipal coroners' courtrooms. If an inquest was considered necessary, it would be held in a local building such as a public house, or a Poor Law workhouse.

What was called 'laying out' the dead was traditionally undertaken by women, occasionally by female family members, but more usually by a local specialist 'handy-woman'. It involved washing and dressing the body, straightening its limbs, making sure the eyes and mouth were closed, often by the use of coins on the eyelids, and a chin-strap to hold up the jaw. The dead would usually be dressed in white, in nightclothes, underclothes, or in a purpose-made shroud. Because people tended to think more about the prac-ticalities of death in advance, burial clothes were often pre-prepared. The point was to prepare the body for its last home, and to ensure that when mourners visited to say their customary last goodbye, the dead person would look decent and properly cared for.

Families were larger than today, and communities more coherent: when news of a death spread, people would travel miles to pay their last respects. When they saw the corpse for the last time, they would often touch or kiss it, as a final farewell gesture which was believed to help prevent haunting. Verification of death by these means reassured the living that death really had taken place, and served also to help natural grief processes by preventing denial.

Coffins were bespoke and made by a local carpenter who would have measured the body for the coffin, into which he would later help lift the corpse. He would often also provide trestles for the coffin to rest on. It was important to keep its contents cool, as there was no refrigeration, so, if possible it would be kept in a darkened room (blinds down, curtains closed) on the cold side of a house. Such attentions would have been particularly important in summer, as natural decomposition sets in soon after death: warmth must be avoided, or unpleasant odours can develop. Sometimes, the coffin would be covered with a pall, usually a heavy black cloth hired from the carpenter. It served as an insulator to keep the body cool, if possible, and would also help make a new coffin look less stark. The colours appropriate to the pall covering it had their own traditions: a child or unmarried teenager, or a poor mother who had died in childbirth, might have a white cloth or sheet for a pall. Even today, children's coffins are often white or pastel in colour. Household fires would be extinguished, and clocks were traditionally stopped when a dead body lay in the house.

Watching the dead can be dated with certainty at least to the fourteenth century. People tried not to leave the body alone. It was considered a duty to 'watch' the dead day and night: very bad to desert them. Families shared this task, which derived from a sense that between death and burial the body had needs, one of which was to be kept company. No one could be quite certain what happened to the dead person's spirit, and there was a feeling that in the interval between death and burial it might still be about. Windows would be opened to allow it to escape, and mirrors and other reflective surfaces were covered, apparently to prevent it becoming trapped. Such customs express fear of haunting. Ghost stories were certainly in wide circulation and belief in death omens widespread. Many customs had an edge of superstition or folk belief about them. One was that the corpse of a murdered person would bleed afresh if the murderer came within its vicinity, which suggests that even when dead, the body was believed to possess some kind of awareness, sensibility or sentience.

Watching the body may also have expressed a hopeful fear that the dead might return to life, and require assistance. There were no sophisticated tests for death, families listened for a heartbeat, and looked for other signs of life: a feather might detect air movement near the mouth, or a mirror condensation. Some are said to have placed a saucer of salt on the chest: salt has many allegorical and spiritual connotations, and its tiny crystals might serve to register movement. Stories circulated about dead people sitting up in their coffins, and doubtless this was a more common experience in days when the fact of death was simple to ascertain, but easy to get wrong. Even today, stories emerge in the papers from time to time of people waking up in the mortuary, after having been taken for dead.

The best safeguard that death really had taken place was in the observance of traditional care of the dying, which could involve various acceptable ways of 'easing' a slow and painful death, and waiting for the sound of the death-rattle of the last breaths, now known as Cheyne-Stokes breathing. The long interval between death and burial, a week, on average, allowed funerary arrangements to be finalized, and funding raised, as well as providing time for distant relatives to receive news and travel to pay their last respects, a custom still extant today. It also served to reassure everyone by confirming the reality of death.

Many customs associated with the dead (like the salt) had resonances both physical and symbolic: the washing of the body could be taken as a figurative cleansing of sins; white burial clothes were associated with innocence. It was traditional to place refreshments near the body, as much as for the dead as for the living. Funerary refreshments, too, had multiple meanings: for example, special biscuits would be served at funerals in willow baskets; willow is associated with water, and sorrow, and also with folk medicine (willow contains analgesic and antiseptic compounds – aspirin is a derivative). In one well-recorded case, a teetotal visitor, who had declined the traditional glass of wine beside the corpse, was urged: 'But you must drink, sir. It's like the Sacrament. It's to kill the sins of my sister' (Leather 1912: 121). Such an entreaty suggests the powerful penumbra of folk religion present in the death chamber.

The body buried in the sure and certain hope of a glorious resurrection was to await the last trumpet which would sound on the Last Day. Taking the words of the burial service as gospel, many people believed, and many more hoped, that the actual body laid in the grave would eventually be changed, to rise up to meet its maker. The churchyard dead, lying safely at rest, sustained communities near and far in the comforting hope of future reunion.

Far more could be said about the death culture of the British Isles, but the point of this brief synopsis is to demonstrate that death tapped into deep wells of custom and belief, and that appropriate care of the dead was held to assure both the future repose of the soul *and* the comfort of mourners (Richardson 2000).

Exploring anatomy and the rise of the bodysnatchers

Readers will perhaps appreciate what a shock it must have been to those in the early stages of mourning to discover that bodysnatchers had been at work: that a dear relative or friend, for whom all the proper observances had been followed, had been rudely turfed out of their long home and stolen away in the dead of night. Such discoveries were not rare in Britain in the Georgian era (1714–1830), particularly in districts within reach of a medical school. A fresh body meant fresh grief. A corpse was at its most valuable for the teaching of anatomy, and hence to the bodysnatchers, when survivors were at their most vulnerable.

To understand bodysnatching and its long legacy into our own time, we have now to look at the history of anatomy. The tuition of anatomy by dissection has historically been, and remains, a crucial element in medical education and training, particularly of surgeons. Recognizing this, government has historically sought to supply colleges of surgery and medicine with corpses on which to teach. In the time of Henry VIII in the sixteenth century, dissection was made a judicial punishment reserved for the worst of murderers. At first, annual grants of bodies were small, no more than a handful a year; but as time passed, the professions pressured government to increase supply. In the mid-eighteenth century, dissection was made a legitimate part of the death sentence in all cases of murder.

Public hangings in the Georgian era were celebrated as a sort of carnival, in which the criminal played an active part, traditionally dressing in white, making a speech from the gallows, acting 'game' to the end, and perhaps plotting with friends and family to be cut down before fully dead, and rushed off to be revived (Linebaugh 1977, 1991). Rare cases were reported in which revival attempts succeeded, so those hanged for lesser crimes may have entertained comforting hopes of rescue. Being sentenced to dissection, however, denied any such hope to murderers, and moreover destroyed any comfort the condemned might otherwise have entertained concerning their own burial, after the execution was over. The law stated that in no case whatsoever was the body of any murderer to be buried.

As a post-mortem punishment, dissection served a complex role in retributive justice. It provided a significant element in the theatre of public execution. As an abhorrent additional punishment, dissection promised the exposure of nakedness, dismemberment and the deliberate destruction of the corpse: a process described in statute law as a *further Terror and peculiar Mark of Infamy*. Dissection represented a gross assault on the integrity and the identity of the body, and upon the repose of the soul, each of which (in other circumstances) would traditionally have been carefully nurtured.

Dissection promised not only the retribution of a fate worse than death:

it served judicially to distinguish the punishment of murder from other capital crimes. Moreover, it provided corpses for the medical Colleges to dissect, and publicly demonstrated the bond cementing the medical profession and the Crown. Dissection was a bitterly unpopular punishment, highly successful because of its flagrant contravention of traditional care of the dead, from the early Tudor era almost to the Britain of Queen Victoria. The bodies of the hanged designated for dissections were protected at the gallows by the full force of the law: preserved to ensure their physical and spiritual obliteration (Linebaugh 1977, 1991).

The Georgian artist, William Hogarth, drew a scene showing a murderer's body being officially dissected at one of the Royal Colleges in London (Richardson 2000). In *The Four Stages of Cruelty* (1751), the noose remains knotted around the dead man's neck, and his bowels and heart have already been extracted by an anatomist, who is shown reaching inside the ribcage for more. The dead man's eye is being poked out by an assistant, a dog sniffs at his heart (which lies on the floor in the foreground) and another assistant rummages in a bucket of entrails. The medical audience looks on, as a lector reads descriptions of the parts from a text, and the presiding chairman, seated high on a dais (under a crest emphasizing the healing art), points with a long stick towards the parts being described.

The conventional manner of teaching anatomy by rote had become increasingly old-fashioned by Hogarth's day. William Harvey (who famously described the circulation of the blood in 1628) had dissected the bodies of his own father and sister, a very enterprising and unusual form of body procurement. In Britain's major towns, private medical schools began opening their doors to provide anatomy tuition to would-be medical men. Reading, pointing and rote-learning was out: teaching was by hands-on dissection.

The number of people hanged for murder was known to be insufficient to supply the growing numbers of students dissecting in these private schools. Complaints about the shortage of corpses became progressively more vocal as the eighteenth century progressed. The Act of Parliament granting the bodies of all murderers to the doctors (25 Geo. 11c.37, 1752) did not significantly alleviate the problem. Medical demand had long outstripped the legal supply. Official medical and surgical examinations were at first tacitly and later openly based on the understanding that extra-legal bodies were being dissected outside College premises, and that corpses beyond the legal provision were being used. Resort was being made to bodysnatching.

At first, students had gone out to dig at night in burial grounds to obtain corpses for themselves, but as the public became aware of what was happening, this activity became more dangerous. Demand promoted supply, giving rise to a class of entrepreneurs whom we know as bodysnatchers, grave-robbers, or 'resurrectionists'. Anatomy schools paid these men well to accept the risks of procurement: their earnings were many times the skilled working wage. As the public became better informed as to how to preserve their dead from predation, prices rose: in times of shortage rising to 20 guineas per corpse. Schools covered costs by selling body parts on to students at a profit. Teaching anatomy in the Georgian era depended to a great extent on the ability of the human body to be bought and sold, or, as the economists describe it, attain commodity value, rather along the lines of butchers' meat. This was a market economy of goods and services: the services involved teaching and practice on the goods, and the goods bought and sold were human corpses and their parts.

Corpses were priced up, haggled over, negotiated for, discussed in terms of supply and demand, delivered, imported, exported and transported. Human bodies were compressed into boxes, packed in sawdust, packed in hay, trussed up in sacks, roped up like hams, sewn in canvas, packed in cases, casks, barrels, crates and hampers, salted, pickled, and injected with pre- servative. They were carried in carts and wagons, in steamboats and barrows, manhandled, damaged in transit, hidden under loads of vegetables. They were stored in cellars and on quays. Human bodies were dismembered and sold in pieces, or measured and sold by the inch. A Lambeth gang was said to have sold adult corpses for 'two guineas and a crown' while children's were sold for 'six shillings for the first foot, and nine (pence) per inch for all it measures more in length' (Richardson 2000: 57). A stolen body's destiny was common knowledge: immediate sale to those who would dismember and obliterate it, like the corpse of a murderer.

Bodysnatching negated traditional death culture, tormented the dying and denied the bereaved imaginative comfort. It nullified their efforts to ensure peaceful rest for the dead. It deprived the dead of their rightful place in the grave, and the future prepared for them, and it deprived survivors of the comfort of knowing where to commune with them. Grave robbery mangled grief processes by compounding these deprivations with the ominous threat of haunting, and ruptured hopes of companionable resurrection.

Perhaps it is not surprising, then, to hear that in cases where body- snatching was discovered, entire communities would vehemently confront the matter. In early 1795, for example, the parishioners of the village of Lambeth (on the south bank of the River Thames facing Westminster) heard that three men had been caught leaving their parish burial ground, carrying five bodies in sacks:

> in consequence of such a discovery, people of all descriptions, whose relatives had been buried in that Ground, resorted thereto, and de- manded to dig for them ... being refused, they in great numbers forced their way in, and in spight of every effort the parish Officers could use, began like Mad people to tear up the ground. [Many empty coffins were found.] Great Distress and agitation of mind was

manifest in every one, and some, in a kind of phrensy, ran away with the coffins of their deceased relations.

(Dopson 1949: 69)

A particularly well-documented instance, dating from 1818, records similar scenes of collective distress in the United States, which shows that this kind of spontaneous cultural response to grave robbery was not confined to the UK (Crowell 1818; Sappol 2002; Richardson 2004).

Opposition to bodysnatching was widespread. The wealthy went to considerable lengths to obtain multiple coffins and secure burial vaults, while entire parishes would club together to pay for churchyard lighting, watchmen or ingenious equipment to thwart the grave-robbers. In poor districts, clubs were formed to share the duty of watching the graveyard. The simplest expedient, resorted to by the very poor, was the use of straw mixed in with the earth returned to the grave, to choke the snatchers' shovels. Occasionally full-scale riots erupted, resulting in attacks on doctors' houses, and the complete demolition of anatomy schools (Richardson 2004).

The Georgian father of transplant surgery

Although transplantation is often thought of as a modern approach in surgery, it has long historical roots. The place of John Hunter, the famous eighteenth-century surgeon-anatomist in the transplant narrative is genuine and verifiable. Hunter was steeped in dissection, experimentation and research into the grafting of tissue. He ran a private medical school and was the recipient of bodysnatched corpses. Hunter is regarded by many as a founding father of transplantation, in a scientific sense. He successfully transplanted a cockerel's spur from its heel to the site of the comb on its head (Hunter 1778). The graft took, and Hunter made a specimen of it, so physical evidence of the transplant's success survived both the cockerel's (and later, Hunter's own) demise.

It is now recognized that Hunter's operation on the cockerel succeeded because the transplanted tissue derived from the cockerel itself, and so was not rejected by the bird's immune system. It was what we would now refer to as an 'auto' (self) transplant. Hunter is said to have also successfully swapped body parts *between* animals. Not all his attempts worked, but there were enough successes to encourage him to continue: they are now thought to have succeeded because they were between siblings, or those with some other close genetic relationship which served to prevent or delay tissue rejection. One so far unexplained success concerns the transplant into a cockerel's comb of a fresh human tooth. Hunter also developed the idea of transplanting tissue in humans. The story is uncomfortable and reflects badly on him, which perhaps explains why it is seldom raised. Since it embroiled Hunter in grim public controversy that led to a suspension of interest in transplantation for several generations, it ought to be better known.

The success of the cockerel auto-transplants led Hunter to try the experiment of transplanting human teeth (Hunter 1778). The initial impetus may simply have been the reinstatement of teeth extracted in error, or knocked out by some accident (i.e. auto-transplant). Hunter however soon tried using *other* sources of human teeth to replace rotten ones (i.e. cosmetic surgery). Initially, he probably tried teeth from the freshly dead corpses secretly delivered to his school of anatomy by bodysnatchers, but before long, he was advocating the use of live transplants. It all sounded quite logical:

> The spurs of the young cock can be made to grow on his [own] comb, or on that of another cock, and its testicles, after having been removed, may be made to unite to the inside of any cavity of another animal . . . Teeth after having been drawn and inserted into the sockets of another person, unite to the new socket, which is called *transplanting*. The engrafting of trees succeeds upon the same principle.
>
> (Hunter 1778)

This short passage is weighty with significance. Most conspicuous, perhaps, is the extraordinary leap from animal experiment to human application, a leap evidently not merely intellectual, but actual. The passage discloses Hunter's complete innocence of any conception of incompatibility: it would be a century and a half before Peter Medawar's outstanding work on the notion of tissue rejection (Fox and Swazey 2002).

Hunter's use of horticultural terms, too, is noteworthy. Indeed, he may have been the first to use the term 'transplanting' for the transposition of tissue from person to person. Hunter may have been drawn to such imagery as it allowed him to minimize, normalize and render unobjectionable the extraction of healthy teeth from one person for cosmetic dentistry in another. His horticultural language echoes in our own time, and for similar reasons, in terminology such as the 'harvesting' of human organs.

In the first flush of his enthusiasm in the 1770s, Hunter assumed that teeth transplanted in this way would last for years, recommending the use of *young second teeth*, freshly extracted from mouths of children. He urged having several children ready, so that if the first tooth didn't fit well into the recipient's socket, others could be tried instead. High-class dentists rapidly adopted the method, which became a fashionable vogue.

Medical ethics was not an established discipline at that time (that, too, would take another 150 years). No ethical committees existed to discuss or legislate on such matters. If a wealthy patient was eager for such treatment, and a practitioner had no conscience, there was nothing to prevent the offer of cash for children's teeth. The lack of ethical committees to discuss or legislate upon such matters, however, did not mean no ethical oversight existed. Among contemporaries who recognized and criticized the horror of Hunter's activities was the novelist Helenus Scott, who related the tales of poor children rendered toothless by the age of 12: their perfect early second teeth extracted to improve the appearance of people of 'quality': ' "My sister," replied the boy, "is much worse off than I am. It is but a poor comfort to her that her teeth are at Court, while she lives at home on slops, without any hope of a husband" ' (Anon. (Scott, H) 1782).

The great caricaturist Thomas Rowlandson published a caricature, *Transplanting of Teeth* (1787), showing a surgeon-dentist and his assistant busily at work transplanting teeth. Rowlandson's dentist advertises his social connections with a royal warrant: 'Dentist to her High Mightyness the Empress of Russia', while another poster reveals the incentive offered 'Most Money Given for Live Teeth'. The cartoon's censure was directed at the wealthy beneficiaries of the operation and their assiduous agents, the surgeons. Both are shown as vain and contemptible exploiters of poverty (Richardson 1999). The child victim-donors (*there is still no satisfactory term for people coerced by poverty into selling their own body-parts*) are shown in rags. A young girl holds her jaw, as she gazes at the small coin she has been paid.

Both Scott (1782) and Rowlandson (1787) seem to have recognized what Hunter ignored: the immorality of his actions. They discerned the profound venality of the transaction, and exposed it to public scrutiny: the catastrophic long-term effects upon children, already poor, of the removal of healthy second teeth; the dietary impact of being unable to masticate, as well as the serious damage to facial appearance, resulting in the likely loss of opportunity for a normal married or working life. Above all, they held up for public reproach the deeply exploitative axis of surgeon/rich client *versus* poor child. The central figure in Rowlandson's image is a chimney-sweep, a notoriously vulnerable figure in eighteenth-century England. Climbing boys were usually parish orphans, known to lack protection from cruel and rapacious employers, who sometimes forced them out to beg if work was scarce.

Tooth transplants were at first hailed as exciting new research findings ready for application in the real world (Hunter 1778). When it became evident that transplanted teeth didn't last, inflammation was invariably followed by decomposition of the teeth, they began to be regarded askance. Although he did not know it, Hunter's efforts were confounded by the body's immune system, which (unless taken from the self or from an identical twin) recognizes a graft as 'other' and rejects it, much as it serves to defend the body from a disease. Then, in 1785, Hunter was confronted with another, and fatal, danger of his over-enthusiasm. A society physician reported in the medical press the horrible death of a young woman from syphilis, conveyed in a transplanted tooth (Watson 1785; Richardson 1999).

Hunter seems to have been impervious to ethical criticism. Despite mounting evidence, he continued to cast doubt on stories of disease spread, and to deny clinical failure. How any doctor could have failed to recognize the long-term damage to the child 'donors' is difficult to see. John Hunter had expert knowledge of the anatomy of childhood dentition, and if his logic allowed tissue to transplant effectively, why not also disease? This unwillingness to look directly at the real consequences of this type of surgical intervention, I have elsewhere termed *'Hunter's blindness'*: the ability to focus so narrowly on recipient-benefit as to excise the humanity of the donor from contemplation (Richardson 2000).

Hunter's work on tissue grafts brought the idea into disrepute, and did not therefore lead directly to the development of transplantation in the modern era. His transplantation work is nevertheless highly significant because, when properly understood in context, it yields a much deeper understanding of the field. Hunter encountered a number of scientific and ethical problems, some of which have dogged the study of anatomy and experimental surgery ever since (see Box 1.1).

Box 1.1 John Hunter and transplantation

Hunter:

- employed agents to obtain human bodies and body parts by theft or subterfuge;
- used animals, human corpses and living human individuals for experimental and commercial transplants;
- exemplifies the phenomenon of unwarranted surgical alacrity;
- understood the need for freshness of transplanted tissue and of matching for size, both of which have been found key to the success of modern organ transplantation;
- encountered graft rejection and disease spread, recognizing neither;
- paid inducements to living 'donors' who were unprotected minors;
- knew the direction of benefit was from poor children to rich adults;
- violated the central Hippocratic dictum 'Above all, do no harm';
- was apparently impervious to ethical criticism;
- is admired and eulogized by many who are ignorant of these matters, since negative aspects of his work are usually edited out or glossed over.

The Anatomy Act

During Hunter's lifetime and beyond, despite all the public's ingenuity in defending the grave by a multitude of security measures, dissecting rooms were still supplied, whether by bribery or sheer nerve. Prices for bodies rose inexorably, offering greater incentives to bodysnatchers, but eventually driving students to decamp abroad to study, which of course affected the profitability of existing medical schools. Everybody was vulnerable to predation: bodies were being taken from the coffins of every social class, countrywide. Ultimately, in 1828, the joint chorus of shortage from the medical schools and pain and anger from the bereaved succeeded in prompting Parliament to establish a Select Committee of the House of Commons to investigate the matter. John Hunter's famous pupil Sir Astley Cooper provided those investigating with a succinct account of the pricing mechanism for corpses, the greater the difficulty of procurement, the higher the price: 'There is no person, let his situation in life be what it may, whom if I were disposed to dissect, I could not obtain. The law only enhances the price, and does not prevent the exhumation' (Cooper 1828).

By the 1820s, the problem had become so public and so extraordinarily contentious, that individuals were coming forward to donate their bodies to medical schools. Although some of these people were candid disbelievers in religious orthodoxies, like Jeremy Bentham, others were not (Richardson and Hurwitz 1987; Richardson 2000). Diverse suggestions were put to the House of Commons Select Committee on Anatomy as to how a safe and unobjectionable supply of corpses for anatomy might be obtained by legislation. Ideas ranged from the need for prominent exemplars to make body donation acceptable, or fashionable (the exemplary person most often proposed was the king), to the dissection of all suicides, all hanged criminals, all those dying in prisons (where death-rates were high), importation from abroad, or the offer of money rewards for future donations.

It swiftly became evident, however, that the Select Committee was not really interested in promoting the idea of consented donation. Its collective mind was already set upon an altogether different expedient. When the Committee's Report was published, it proposed a new Act of Parliament to provide a new source of corpses so cheap and easily available that it would undermine the bodysnatchers' market economy. Murderers would no longer be dissected. All those who died in poverty, without money enough for a funeral, would henceforth be liable to be taken for dissection. The proposal would transfer a much hated and feared punishment for murder to poverty. The idea suited the dominant politics of the day, which was strongly in favour of cutting public expenditure by penalizing poverty (Richardson 2000).

The Members of Parliament on the Select Committee were oblivious to the fact that two men in Edinburgh had already hit upon an even more profitable method of corpse procurement. Before and during the hearing of evidence from people like Sir Astley Cooper, and while the Report of the Committee's deliberations was being drafted and printed, ten people had already met their deaths. More would die at the hands of Burke and Hare before their last murder, on Halloween 1828, and their capture the following day (Dudley Edwards 1993; Richardson 2000).

Famous today as bodysnatchers, Burke and Hare in fact never robbed a grave. They obtained corpses by offering hospitality to people down on their luck, plying them with drink and smothering them as they slept. Their bodies were sold to an anatomy school in Edinburgh run by Dr Robert Knox, who approved their freshness, and asked no questions as to how they had been obtained (Richardson 2000). These bodies were not more than a day old, and had never been laid out, so there certainly should have been serious suspicions. The generous cash paid and medical unconcern about the corpses' derivation encouraged Burke and Hare to continue.

They were caught not by medical discernment of signs of foul play upon the bodies supplied, but by suspicious neighbours. Because most of the physical evidence of their handiwork had already been destroyed in the dissecting room, Hare was offered legal immunity from prosecution in exchange for evidence against his accomplice. Burke eventually confessed to the deaths of 16 people. Hare went free, and Burke was hanged and dissected, one of the last cohort of murderers to undergo that fate (Richardson 2000).

The case caused a national furore of fear and anger, which became known as 'burkophobia'. After the discovery of a new series of murders by copycat criminals in London in 1831 (Bishop and Williams, thought to have dispatched over 50 people) burkophobia served to hasten the passage of the Anatomy Act through Parliament in 1832, despite considerable opposition to its punitive effect upon the poor (Richardson 2000).

The Anatomy Act effectively decreed that the destitute were to be dissected in the name of scientific progress. It is true to say that the Act had an 'opt-out' facility, on this Parliament and the public had been reassured. The Act stated that the poor could choose not to be dissected by swearing to this fact before two witnesses. But the opt-out clause was unenforceable inside a Poor Law workhouse, where the only witnesses were as powerless as the dead.

Fear of dying in the workhouse so terrified the Victorian poor and their children that they contributed vast profits to the big insurance companies by paying in their millions for penny-a-week policies to cover funeral costs. The pauper funeral became the signature of social failure, and helps explain why a 'decent' funeral in Victorian and even early twentieth-century Britain provided so visible a public display, and why even in recent times, a pauper's funeral was regarded as something to be avoided at all costs (Richardson 1988).

The Anatomy Act was not, as had been hoped, the hoped-for remedy for the shortage of teaching material. Victorian medical schools suffered from chronic shortages of bodies on which to teach, because not only did the poor do everything they could to save themselves from being coerced into the pauper's fate, but those people who might have been willing to become donors believed their gift was no longer needed. Shortage of human dissection material dogged the teaching of anatomy right up to the Second World War. At that time, most of those dissected in medical schools were being taken from the mortuaries of mental institutions (Richardson 2000).

The growth of voluntary donation

Change occurred only in the mid-twentieth century, and in parallel with a genuinely significant change of government attitude towards the sick poor, made publicly manifest in the creation of the new NHS in 1948. For the first time in UK history, there evolved equilibrium between the number of bodies freely available and the number required for teaching and research. The Anatomy Act remained in force, virtually unaltered since 1832. These bodies were, and are, provided, in a spirit of trust and generosity, by voluntary public donation (Richardson 2000). There was no change in the law until the introduction of the Human Tissue Act (2004) legislation that covers the removal, storage and use of human organs and other tissue for scheduled purposes (see Appendix 1).

Who these early donors were is not known, as no study of UK whole-body donors was published until 1995. Nevertheless the first survey provides helpful indications as to what sort of people do donate, and why (Richardson and Hurwitz 1995). They were not easy to categorize generationally (age range = 19–95), socially (various) or in terms of religious belief (various/none), but the reasons they gave for their wish to donate their own bodies for dissection were altruistic, and quite fiercely antagonistic to any suggestion of financial or other reward. Many envisaged the benefits of their donation would flow to 'future patients', 'mankind', and 'Joe Public', so their impulse seems to have been both egalitarian and philanthropic.

The twentieth century witnessed a rise in other forms of bodily donation, too. The development of blood transfusion services in wartime probably influenced the public's willingness to donate bodies for dissection, and this rise in bodily generosity, in turn, meant that when organ transplantation became feasible in the optimistic period following the Second World War, there were people willing to come forward to donate their own or their relatives' organs to save other people's lives. Of course, not everyone was willing, but the evidence points towards a proportion of the population to whom bodily generosity of this sort was not objectionable. It is highly significant that 47 per cent of the whole-body donors surveyed were or had been blood donors, and 63 per cent of them carried organ donor cards; twice the national average for a comparable group at that time (Richardson and Hurwitz 1995).

The numbers of individuals currently registering a wish to donate organs in the UK by joining the NHS Organ Donor Register, in the ten years of its existence, stands at 13,461,986; 22 per cent of the population (UK Transplant 2006). Those who find themselves in the predicament of having to ponder the matter of giving a relative's organs are more often reluctant to agree because they feel their relative has already suffered enough and they wish them to remain whole and not to be cut (Sque *et al.* 2006). This notion reveals the fear that the removal of body parts may involve additional suffering for the individual, which reveals a close kinship between thought processes today and those of the past in which the corpse was believed to possess some sort of sentience after death. Older beliefs and customs form the bedrock of our current death traditions. We still want the body presented decently; and although church attendance has declined and Christian belief waned, there remains the nebulous hope of future reunification and a profound repugnance towards physical interference or mutilation after death.

Conclusion

In this chapter I have tried to offer a succinct analysis of the historical background so as to assist thinking and debate about some difficult issues in modern transplantation.

For centuries (1540s–1830s) there existed a fragile public acceptance that murderers might legitimately be dissected. The Anatomy Act of 1832 transferred that punishment from murder to poverty. I have tried to show why folk memory resonates with tales of bodysnatching, medical murder and the indignity of dying in poverty. Concern for the dead indicates a sense that the dead have needs. A deep cultural stratum of very old beliefs seems to indicate that the treatment of the dead is held somehow to reflect or affect the fate of the soul.

The history of transplantation itself is rooted in the era of bodysnatching. The healthy second teeth John Hunter extracted from unprotected minors for cosmetic transplantation into the mouths of his wealthy clients were perceived by commentators at the time to have been procured unethically. Repugnance towards the procurement process, the furore concerning iatrogenic spread of fatal diseases, and medical failure, together scotched development of the field for several generations.

We may regard ourselves as truly fortunate that the days are past when these things were commonplace. Yet we cannot altogether ignore news stories from the developing world which document analogous ways in which the very poor remain vulnerable, like London street children in Hunter's day, to the offer of money for body-parts (Scheper-Hughes 2000).

Some doctors and likely transplant patients who perceive remedies for serious bodily ills in transplantation often pressure government and media for still higher levels of organ procurement. It would be well for them to bear in mind that while encouraging donation is one thing, forcing it is quite another: one which risks damaging irrevocably the progress already achieved.

If we may learn anything from the past, it is that medical alacrity should be tempered with humanity and wisdom, and that legislators should keep a keen eye on the likely negative impacts of their efforts. Legislators and medical professionals hoping to encourage public trust and promote bodily donation may find the 1832 Anatomy Act's unenforceable opt-out clause an exemplary cautionary tale: 'presuming' upon the consent of others is not the panacea it may seem to some. The 1832 Act did *not* promote bodily donation. Nor did it supply sufficient bodies for dissection. While it may have strongly encouraged unnecessary funerary expenditure in the Victorian era, the Act did nothing at all to encourage public trust in doctors.

That some of the patients of the new NHS and their children choose to become organ and body donors in the half century after the NHS was established is a remarkable tribute to their own cultural adjustment, and to that of the Service itself, which had to live down a great deal of imputation, as well as the fears which spawned it.

It is my hope that this chapter will serve to remind those who read it about the generosity of organ donors and their families, and to remind us all *never* to take it for granted.

Note

1   Readers wishing to access the detailed research which underlies this chapter are urged to refer to Richardson, R. (2000) *Death, Dissection and the Destitute*, 2nd edn. Chicago: University of Chicago Press, where the history sources are given in much greater detail than is possible here. This chapter has been adapted from Richardson, R. (2006) Human dissection organ donation: a historical social background, *Mortality*, 11(2): 152–65.

References

25 Geo. 11 c.37 (1752) *An Act for Better Preventing the Horrid Crime of Murder*. London: HM Government.

Anon. (Scott, H) (1782) *Adventures of a Rupee*. London: Murray.

Cooper, A. (1828) Evidence, in *Report and Evidence of the Select Committee on Anatomy*. London: HM Government.

Crowell, R. (1818) *A Sermon*. Andover: Flagg Gould.

Dopson, L. (1949) St. Thomas's parish vestry records and a body-snatching incident, *British Medical Journal*, 2: 69.

Dudley Edwards, O. (1993) *Burke and Hare*. Edinburgh: Mercat.

LIVERPOOL JOHN MOORES UNIVERSITY
LEARNING SERVICES

Fox, R. and Swazey, J. (2002) *Spare Parts: Organ Replacement in American Society*, 2nd edn. New Brunswick, NJ: Transaction Publishers.

Higginson, I.J. and Sen-Gupta, G.J.A. (2000) Place of care in advanced cancer a qualitative systematic literature review of patient preferences, *Journal of Palliative Medicine*, 3: 287–300.

Human Tissue Act (2004) London: HMSO.

Hunter, J. (1778) *Natural History of the Human Teeth*. London: Johnson.

Leather, E.M. (1912) *The Folklore of Herefordshire*. London: Sidgwick & Jackson.

Linebaugh, P. (1977) The Tyburn riot against the surgeons, in D. Hay, P. Linebaugh, J.G. Rule, E.P. Thompson and C. Winslow (eds) *Albion's Fatal Tree: Crime and Society in Eighteenth Century England*. London: Penguin.

Linebaugh, P. (1991) *The London Hanged*. London: Allen Lane.

Redfern, M. (2001) *The Royal Liverpool Children's Inquiry Report*. London: The Stationery Office.

Richardson, R. (1988) The nest-egg and the funeral: fear of death on the parish among the elderly, in A. Gilmore and S. Gilmore (eds) *A Safer Death: Proceedings of the First International Conference on Multidisciplinary Aspects of Terminal Care, 1988*. London: Plenum Press.

Richardson, R. (1999) Transplanting teeth: reflections on a cartoon by Thomas Rowlandson, *The Lancet*, 354: 1740.

Richardson, R. (2000) *Death, Dissection and the Destitute*, 2nd edn. Chicago: University of Chicago Press.

Richardson, R. (2004) Bodily theft past and present: a tale of two sermons, *The Lancet* (Medicine Crime and Punishment Supplement), 364: 44–5.

Richardson, R. and Hurwitz, B.S. (1987) Jeremy Bentham's self-image: an exemplary bequest for dissection, *British Medical Journal*, 295: 195–8.

Richardson, R. and Hurwitz, B.S. (1995) Donors' attitudes towards body donation for dissection, *The Lancet*, 346: 277–9.

Sappol, M. (2002) *A Traffic of Dead Bodies: Anatomy and Embodied Social Identity in Nineteenth-Century America*. Princeton, NJ: Princeton University Press.

Scheper-Hughes, N. (2000) The global traffic in human organs, *Current Anthropology*, 41: 191–224. See also the OrgansWatch Project at Berkeley: sunsite.berkeley.edu/biotech/organwatch (accessed 6 March 2006).

Sque, M., Long, T., Payne, S. and Allardyce, D. (2006) *Exploring the End of Life Decision-making and Hospital Experiences of Families Who Did Not Donate Organs for Transplant Operations. Final Research Report for UK Transplant*. University of Southampton, Southampton: UK.

UK Transplant (2006) www.uktransplant.org.uk/ukt/default.jsp (accessed 22 July 2006).

Watson, W. (1785) Report of a fatal venereal infection from a transplanted tooth, *Medical Transactions of the Royal Society*, 3: 325–8.

Youngner, S., Fox, R. and O'Connell, L.J. (1996) *Organ Transplantation: Meanings and Realities*. Madison, WI: University of Wisconsin Press.

2 Contemporary views of bereavement and the experience of grief

Sheila Payne

Introduction

It is widely acknowledged that bereavement represents one of the major challenges facing people (Payne *et al.* 1999). But all bereavements are not the same. The nature of the relationship, the stage in life of both the deceased and the bereaved person, the anticipated or unexpected nature of the loss, the nature and reason for the death and the way the dead body is treated all impact on how each loss is experienced and the meaning attributed to it. The starting point of all cadaveric organ donations is the death of another human being and therefore it is essential to understand how loss and bereavement are conceptualized and experienced.

Requests for organ donation are more likely to arise out of sudden, un-expected and untimely deaths (Sque and Payne 1996) and there is evidence that these types of bereavement are even more challenging than those which are anticipated (Stroebe and Schut 2001; Relf 2004). In this situation, family members have little or no time to adjust to the loss. They may struggle to take on the enormity of the events that are unfolding. They therefore cannot experience anticipatory grief which, in expected deaths associated with terminal illness, may allow some rehearsal of how they may manage after the death and an opportunity to develop new skills and interests (Evans 1994). There is evidence that sudden, unexpected deaths that are associated with violence or are perceived as traumatic, such as bleeding to death or drowning, increase the likelihood of grief complications (Stroebe and Schut 2001).

In this chapter I will be arguing that in contemporary western society, there have been a number of discourses that serve to shape understanding of loss and bereavement. In addition, most of the major religions have also provided explanations for loss and accounts of what happens at the time of and after death, which many people find comforting (Parkes *et al.* 1997). The chapter aims to introduce three perspectives on understanding bereavement and to briefly introduce bereavement support interventions. The purpose is to enable readers to understand how conceptual models of loss and bereavement have been influential in shaping contemporary ways to talk and think about grief and behave during bereavement. They also provide a useful way for health and social care professionals to understand the diversity of responses and meanings given to the experience of bereavement. Walter (1999) has, for instance, argued that in contemporary British society assumptions about appropriate grieving and mourning behaviours vary by social class and background.

The three theoretical perspectives will include intra-psychic, inter-personal and social approaches. The work of Freud, Bowlby, Parkes, Worden and Kulber-Ross are examples of stage/phase models of loss that focus on psychological processes, in particular emotional and cognitive processes. Many of these theories have been drawn from psychiatric and psychological clinical experience and research. It will be argued that they have become very influential in guiding grief counselling and other interventions. Newer in-teractional models drawn from the stress and coping literature, including the dual process model will be covered. The third perspective will discuss social aspects of bereavement, including role transitions and the 'continuing bonds' hypothesis. The chapter will end by briefly considering the assumptions that underpin bereavement support and look at the evidence for the effectiveness of bereavement interventions.

It is generally agreed that there are no single 'correct' or 'true' theories which explain the experience of loss or account for the emotions, experiences and cultural practices which characterize grief and mourning (Payne *et al.* 1999; Hockey *et al.* 2001). A postmodern position suggests that individual diversity is paramount, and that within broad cultural constraints, each of us develops our own ways of *doing* bereavement (Walter 1999). Some ways of talking and thinking about bereavement have become so popular that many people are unaware of their origins and they have become part of our taken-for-granted knowledge about bereavement. It is normal for bereave-ment texts to start by defining key terms such as bereavement, grief and mourning (Stroebe *et al.* 2001) but as will be argued these very terms arise out of particular ways to construe bereavement. As explained by Payne *et al.* (1999), the common root of the words bereavement and grief (reave) are derived from the Old English word 'reafian', to plunder, spoil or rob, so the sense of personal violation and the heaviness of the soul are embedded in the language itself. *Bereavement* is usually defined as the process surrounding the loss of a loved object. In the context of this chapter, this is a person who has died and is being considered as suitable for organ donation. The bereaved person's reaction to this loss is described as *grief*. Anthropologists and others have long debated whether grief is a universal human response to bereave-ment and loss. *Mourning* is generally described as the behavioural, emotional and cognitive expression of grief. Mourning is heavily influenced by cultural, age and gender specific norms. For example, in some cultures women do not attend funerals or in the past dead newborns were not afforded a separate grave. While it may appear simple and straightforward to separate out these aspects of loss into neat definitions, Small (2001) has argued that they are intimately linked to our theoretical understanding of loss. So the concepts and language we use to describe bereavement both reveal and shape our understanding of this experience.

Discourses of bereavement

Intra-psychic perspectives

Perhaps the most influential understandings of loss and bereavement throughout the last century have arisen from psychological and psychiatric perspectives, which have focused on the intra-psychic domain. They have emphasized how people think and especially how they feel, their emotions. They prioritize the internal mental dialogues which occur inside people's heads; the rumination, dwelling upon and thinking about the loss which has come to be called 'grief work'. For many people, especially health and social care workers, these models have become so popular that it is now regarded as taken for granted that bereavement is like this. No historical account can be complete without reference to the seminal work of Freud.

Writing at the time of the First World War (1914–18) when many European countries were overwhelmed by the tragic loss of life among their young men, Freud (1917) pointed out the similarities and differences between grief and depression in his classic text *Mourning and Melancholia*. His paper offered one of the first accounts of normal and pathological grief. The thoughts discussed in it underpin his psychoanalytic theory of depression and provide the base for many current theories of grief and its resolution. In the light of the impact of Freud's theory of grief on subsequent theoretical developments, it is surprising to acknowledge that grief as a psychological process was never Freud's main focus of interest. In the paper, he argued that people become attached to others who are important for the satisfaction of their needs and to whom emotional expression is directed. Love is conceptualized as the attachment of emotional energy to the psychological representation of the loved person. It is assumed that the more important the relationship, the greater the degree of attachment. According to Freudian theory, grieving represents a dilemma because there is a simultaneous need to relinquish the relationship so that the person may regain the energy invested and a wish to maintain the bond with the love object. The individual needs to accept the reality of the loss so that the emotional energy can be released and redirected. The process of withdrawing energy from the lost object is called 'grief work'. Freud regarded this intra-psychic processing as essential to the breaking of relationship bonds with the deceased, to allow the reinvestment of emotional energy and the formation of new relationships with others. Freud's most important contributions to understanding bereavement have been:

- introducing a developmental perspective in which grief is seen as a process to be accomplished over time;
- introducing the notion of 'grief work' which he regarded as effortful and time-consuming;
- delineating the difference between grief and depression.

Freud's ideas were expanded upon and developed by others, most notably by John Bowlby, a British psychiatrist. They have provided the foundation for a lot of subsequent theoretical developments and therapeutic interventions. In the second half of the twentieth century, Bowlby (1969, 1973, 1980) proposed a complex theory of attachment to account for the formation of close human relationships, especially between mothers and their babies, and for what happened when these bonds were broken. Attachment behaviours are biologically-based behaviours triggered in times of threat which lead to individuals seeking physical proximity with attachment figures. These behaviours therefore have survival functions, as they draw mothers to their infants and vice versa as infants become more mobile. Bowlby's theory offers an evolutionary account of attachment and loss. In the context of organ donation, where family members may find themselves in difficult and confusing situations that are often perceived as threatening, such as in intensive care units, the theory has strong resonance. Let us therefore look more closely at the conceptual development and implications of attachment theory.

Bowlby proposed that reciprocal interaction processes between mothers and infants provided the basis for attachment. Temporary separation was marked by characteristic behaviours and feelings such as distress (crying), protest (calling and shouting) and searching (looking for the 'lost' person) which usually resulted in the coming together of both people. Separation was thought to be an unpleasant state for infants. Therefore, infants quickly developed behaviours such as crying which brought their mothers nearer to them and other social behaviours such as smiling and later talking or physically clinging to their mother which also served to maintain contact. Children build working models of relationships which allow them to predict behaviours such as their mother responding to their distress calls by picking them up and having a cuddle. Over time these relationships become internalized as mental representations of emotional closeness that could be invoked to provide felt security. So in adulthood people will feel comforted if they have a photograph of one loved one by their hospital bed, for example.

Bowbly argued that the responsiveness of the attachment figure to the child determined the security of the attachment relationship. According to Bowlby, the nature of attachment relationships provide the template for other adult relationships and the failure to form mutually satisfying and stable attachments in childhood is associated with adult psychopathology. He suggested that the nature of distress for infants and young children varied sequentially in the following ways (described as stages), the longer the separation occurred:

- *protest* – marked by anger and loud crying, with constant searching for the lost mother and a hypervigilance anticipating her return;
- *despair* – marked by withdrawal and less vigorous crying;
- *detachment* – marked by an outward display of cheerful behaviour but the child remains emotionally distant.

Based on his clinical knowledge and observations of young children, Bowlby thought that permanent loss, such as bereavement, also triggered these feelings of intense distress and the same immediate behavioural responses of crying, searching, clinging, giving way to despondency, depression and later detachment. Bowlby proposed that the intensity of the grief was related to the closeness of the attachment relationship. For example, he predicted that we would be more distressed by the loss of a parent or sibling than a distant cousin, because we had invested more emotional energy in that relationship. In writing about the experience of loss, Bowlby was careful to emphasize that the phases were not discrete entities and that people may oscillate between phases, although over the course of time it was anticipated that people would move through the phases. The four phases following loss were described by Bowlby (1980: 85) as:

1 Phase of numbing that usually lasts from a few hours to a week and may be interrupted by outbursts of extremely intense distress and/or anger.
2 Phase of yearning and searching for the lost figure lasting some months and sometimes for years.
3 Phase of disorganization and despair.
4 Phase of greater or less degree of reorganization.

Because the experience of loss was related to the type of attachment, Bowlby suggested that 'abnormal' attachment patterns were likely to be associated with 'abnormal' grieving. For example, he noted that relationships which were very unequal, such as highly dependent or domineering ones, were more likely to result in difficulties during bereavement. Like Freud, Bowlby emphasized the emotional aspects of loss and the need to 'work through' the loss (thinking about the experience: 'grief work') to achieve an outcome where there was no longer any emotional investment in the dead person ('letting go'). Bowlby's ideas about attachment have been taken up by obstetric services, for example in encouraging early contact between mothers and babies after birth. His ideas were also influential in the development of Parkes' theories of loss (1972, 1986, 1996).

Parkes, a British psychiatrist, was one of the first people to conduct systematic research into the bereavement experiences of widows. In 1971 he suggested that bereavement should be considered as a major psychosocial transition, which challenged the taken-for-granted world of the bereaved person. He argued that most people think of their world as relatively stable, in which they make assumptions of perceived control. Death, especially sudden death, challenges this, as people have to adapt to changes in relationships and social status (e.g. from being a wife to a widow) and economic circumstances (having less money). He, like Bowlby, proposed that people progress through phases in coming to terms with their loss.

Working at approximately the same time in the USA, Kubler-Ross (1969), a psychiatrist who was heavily influenced by psychoanalytic ideas, proposed a stage model of loss in relation to dying which has been applied to bereavement. This model emphasized changing emotional expression throughout the final period of life. Phase models of grief were used by Worden (1982, 1991, 2001) as the theoretical basis of his therapeutic intervention called 'tasks of mourning'. He suggested that grief was a process not a state and that people needed to work through their reactions to loss to achieve a complete adjustment. Over time, Parkes, Kulber-Ross and Worden have modified and developed their ideas and the above account may give a simplistic rendering of their reasoning and the complexity of their thinking.

Evaluation of intra-psychic models and their application to organ donation contexts

All these theories have been critiqued and challenged because they make the assumption that the experience of grief involves a linear progression through phases, stages or tasks and from which there is an eventual outcome where the distress of grief is no longer experienced (Wortman and Silver 1989; Stroebe *et al.* 2005). Notions of change and process are fundamental and failure to 'move on' or 'progress' gives rise to ideas of being 'stuck'. The theories have largely concentrated their attention on the intra-psychic domain (the inner workings of the mind), and especially the necessity of 'grief work': failure to do this is considered 'abnormal'. Stroebe (1992) challenged some aspects of the 'grief work' hypothesis. While she recognized the cognitive processing element of it, she considered that it was limited because it focused attention on just the loss of the dead person and not all the subsequent changes that are likely to arise for a bereaved person. She also challenged the notion that the lack of cognitive processing was potentially pathological by highlighting psychological research which showed that excessive rumination may also be harmful (Nolen-Hoeksema 2001). So just dwelling upon the loss may not be adaptive. She also argued that part of the experience of bereavement is coming to terms with psychosocial changes. In particular, she criticized the emphasis of the 'grief work' hypothesis on intrapsychic processing and its neglect of interpersonal relationships. A recent review of the evidence concluded there was limited support for the hypothesis (Stroebe *et al.* 2005). Phase models also make an assumption that people have some control over their feelings and thoughts, and these can be accessed through talk, such as during counselling sessions.

Implications of intra-psychic approaches to bereavement for organ donation

Box 2.1 summarizes the key implications of phase and stage models of loss for organ donation. They are helpful to health care professionals because they offer some explanations for the profound distress and disruption seen in some family members. They can also account for the numbness and lack of emotional expression seen in others. The important thing is that communication with people facing the challenge of separation and loss is very likely to be complex because it is difficult for them to process new information, to make decisions and to retain information. Therefore the repeated requests for information about the ill person and the checking and counter-checking of facts with other staff should be considered as normal. Newly-bereaved people may also respond in unexpected ways such as with anger or relief.

Box 2.1 Implications of intra-psychic approaches for organ donation situations

- Provide an explanation of different emotions at time of death and in the immediate aftermath, including shock, numbness, anger, distress.
- Provide an explanation of cognitive disruption in the initial period and why people find it so difficult to make decisions relating to donation.
- The degree of cognitive disruption may also make it difficult to understand new information and people may need information repeated.
- Provide an explanation of behaviours when attachment relationships are threatened such as distress (crying and calling), needing to be near the seriously ill or dying relative, restlessness and difficulty in settling when away from this person.
- Indicate why the loss of certain relationships are more disruptive because of the intensity of the attachment relationship.

- Attachment theory suggests that people have little control over these basic responses to the threat of loss and that it is difficult for them to be reassured by communication from health care professionals.
- Phase models suggest that grief tends to resolve over time and that supportive interventions may help people in making these transitions and in acknowledging the reality of the death.
- The maintenance of confidentiality about recipients and outcomes of the donation is probably based on the idea that to complete their grieving bereaved people need to 'let go' of the deceased and develop new attachment relationships with living people.
- The 'grief work' hypothesis provides an explanation of why family members may continue to seek information and contact with transplantation services or with the hospital team, as they work through and reflect upon the death and reasons for the organ donation decision.

Interactional perspectives

The second perspective also arises from psychological theory but in this account less emphasis is placed upon the state of mind and mental processes and more upon how the individual interacts with others and the ways they construe the situation. These concepts have their foundation in psychological theories of stress and coping, in particular the influential transactional theory proposed by Lazarus and Folkman (1984) and subsequently further developed by Folkman (1997). They argued that any event may be perceived as threatening by an individual, and that individuals cognitively appraise situations to estimate the degree of threat and to mobilize resources to cope with it. The outcome of the appraisal may be that the environment is perceived to be benign and no stress response is activated. Alternatively, the situation may be perceived as threatening and the person then needs to mobilize coping resources: called, not surprisingly, 'coping'. Coping may focus on dealing with the threat directly or may emphasize the emotional response that serves to reduce the feeling of stress. These are called 'problem-focused' and 'emotion-focused' coping. For example, in the context of organ donation, family members may be called to the hospital to see a newly-admitted patient. For most people this situation will be appraised as potentially threatening, unless the family member is already expecting their loved one to be at the hospital, perhaps because they work there. However, for most people, being summoned to a hospital is a worrying and threatening scenario, and coping responses are usually mobilized to deal with the threat. For example, a person might seek social support by asking another family member or friend to accompany them. Alternatively, and sometimes simultaneously, people might try to seek information about the patient or try to reduce their sense of distress and worry by concentrating on recalling how young, fit and healthy their family member is. This theoretical model is useful because it shows that stress is both a physical, psychological and behavioural response and that people differ in what they perceive to be stressful. Most things in our environment are within our abilities to adapt to, but it is those things that challenge this adaptation process which are considered to be stressful (Bartlett 1998).

Stroebe and Schut (1999) further developed these ideas within the context of bereavement, and proposed a dual process model. They suggested that, following a death, people oscillate between 'restoration-focused' coping, which is similar to 'problem-focused' coping, for example by dealing with everyday life, and 'grief-focused' coping, which is similar to 'emotion-focused' coping, for example by expressing their distress. They argue that people move between these two forms of coping with loss, although over time coping responses become progressively more 'restoration-focused'. So in the initial period following bereavement it might be anticipated that most of the coping responses would involve emotional coping, such as crying and talking about the lost person. The response of numbness can be seen as a type of emotion-focused coping by inhibiting the display of distressing emotions. However, very soon bereaved people will need to eat, sleep and undertake some tasks of everyday living, especially if they are caring for others such as children. Activities such as shopping for food and caring for children or pets are all forms of restoration-focused coping. They are of course essential to maintain a healthy life but they also provide a distraction from the intensity of feelings triggered by the loss.

Stroebe and Schut (1999) argue that if bereaved people spend too long on either type of coping it is potentially damaging. For example, if people focus only on their distress they may fail to eat sufficient healthy foods, and alternatively if they merely get on with everyday life they may not acknowledge the emotional impact of their loss and not allow themselves time to be sad and to grieve. From these ideas, Stroebe and her team have developed therapeutic interventions to help people address both types of coping to achieve a balance.

Evaluation of interactional approaches and their application to organ donation contexts

These approaches to understanding loss are helpful because they recognize individual diversity and that humans are constantly interacting with others. In terms of organ donation they suggest that it is helpful to realize that people make appraisals of how threatening their environment is perceived to be. This suggests that in hospitals staff may try to arrange space and places like relatives' rooms which are comfortable, quiet and private, away from the clinical setting. For example, an intensive care unit can seem very frightening with strange sounds, sights and smells which can seem highly threatening to family members but is a normal working environment for staff. The number of different medical teams involved in a patient's care may appear very confusing to family members and dying in this context may appear decontextualized (Seymour 2001). Box 2.2 summarizes the implications of the dual process model for understanding the responses of bereaved people during the process of organ donation.

Box 2.2 Implications of interactional approaches for organ donation situations

- This approach provides explanations why people differ so much in their experience of and reaction to loss of an important person and the request for donation.
- They indicate that bereavement responses are mediated by both internal cognitive appraisals but also the coping resources at individuals' disposal. For example, people with supportive networks or strong beliefs in their own mastery may be better able to respond to the challenges of a sudden loss and a request for organ donation.
- People whose coping is predominately problem-focused may value a lot of information about the process and procedures of donation, the chance to witness neurological testing and involvement in decision-making.
- People whose coping is predominately emotion-focused may value empathetic staff who acknowledge their distress and give them an opportunity to express their emotion and grief.
- Interactional approaches suggest that people oscillate between emotion and problem-focused coping, and this is normal. It is helpful for staff to realize that family members may react to difficult communication about organ donation in different ways during the decision-making process. Even the same person may respond in apparently contradictory ways depending upon their current coping mode.
- Interactional approaches suggest that bereavement interventions can be targeted to help people explore other ways of coping if they become 'stuck' in a particular mode.

Social perspectives

The third group of perspectives is based on the assumption that bereavement impacts not only on how people think and feel, and on the interactions they have, but also that it is fundamentally a social process in which people's position in society is changed. This impacts upon their sense of self as they are both a part of and shaped by the society and culture in which they are situated. Field and Payne (2005) have argued that many health professionals have failed to adequately understand the significance of these changes because they tend to focus on individual reactions to loss, particularly psychology factors. Within the context of organ donation, individual decisions need to be understood within the context of the broader society in which they occur, and how in that culture the body and death are conceptualized must be taken into account (Sque *et al.* 2006). Historians and anthropologists have long illustrated the diversity of expressions of loss, in terms of the rituals associated with death, and the impact that different types of loss may have depending upon social status, age and gender of both the deceased and the bereaved (Richardson 2000). Sociological and anthropological perspectives of bereavement emphasize the changes to social role and social relationships that bereavement precipitates. Social roles are very important in defining identity in most western societies. Identity is usually not fixed but is constantly renegotiated throughout the life span (Giddens 1976). Therefore, social factors such as age, gender, social class and ethnicity all impact on the meaning of loss and the way bereavement is enacted (Field *et al.* 1997; Parkes *et al.* 1997). From this perspective, grief is not merely a set of psychological responses which are largely biologically determined (as presented in the intrapsychic approaches) but patterns of grief and possibilities for its expression are largely influenced by social and cultural factors (Reimers 2001; Field and Payne 2005). It is these social perspectives about loss and bereavement which will be examined next to determine their relevance for organ donation situations.

Often, organ donation may be considered in younger people and children when a sudden death has occurred. Deaths that occur in younger people are almost always regarded as untimely and a tragedy. In developed countries, parents normally assume that they will outlive their children and with small family sizes parents tend to invest heavily in the few children they have. Low rates of infant mortality and the prevention or treatment of many acute medical conditions mean that the probability of babies, children and young people dying is generally very low in most developed countries. There are thus few socially accepted accounts to provide a meaning for these deaths.

According to Riches and Dawson (2000), bereaved family members struggle to find a meaning for the death and differences between family members may give rise to different responses and ways of coping with grief. This may manifest in the ways that families respond to the request for organ donation. There are few agreed social responses to the loss of children in developed countries but it tends to be regarded as highly abnormal and threatening.

Families are complex social structures in which there are reciprocal roles and shared identities that are maintained over time by mutual support, with collective memories and goals (Kissane and Bloch 2002). The death of a child challenges many of the taken-for-granted aspects of everyday family life.

Certain roles, such as being a parent, can only be enacted in the presence of a child, therefore the death of an only child removes the possibility of this social role. Parenting is a highly valued social role from which the individual receives not only personal satisfaction but social esteem from others. Parents generally invest a great deal of themselves in the lives of their children and on the death of the child their role of protector and provider is taken away. During the process of organ donation, parents may feel concerned about giving up treatment 'too early' or have fears about the mutilation of their child's body. The death of a child disrupts their sense of identity, not only because the parent may feel guilt about their failure to prevent the child from dying, but because other people react to them in different ways. The loss of a sibling when family sizes are small leaves a gap which is hard or impossible to fill.

Lofland (1985: 181) argues that contemporary western grief is expressed as it is because of four aspects of modern life:

- a relational pattern which links individuals to a small number of highly significant others;
- a definition of death as personal annihilation and as unusual and tragic except among the aged;
- selves which take very seriously their emotional states; and
- interactional settings which provide rich opportunities to contemplate loss.

She argues that cultural expectations that bereavement should be an intensely personal and distressing experience are perpetuated through influential personal accounts and in the self-help and popular literature which tends to present a psychological and emotional account of grief, based on the intra-psychic perspectives presented earlier.

Contemporary sociological accounts have challenged the assumption that for successful resolution of grief, 'letting go' of the relationship needs to occur (Klass *et al.* 1996; Walter 1996). These theories are based on an assumption that people wish to maintain feelings of continuity and that, even though physical relationships will end at the time of death, these relationships become transformed but remain important within the memory of the individual and community. Walter (1996, 1999) proposed a biographical model of loss in which he suggested that bereaved people seek to create a durable and integrated narrative which describes both the person who has died and the part they played in their lives. He argues that these narratives are socially constructed and that because postmodern societies are so fragmented and compartmentalized, people relate to others in different ways depending upon the social roles they occupy at any one time. Klass *et al.* (1996) also proposed a similar model and examined this in relation to different types of loss. They argued that for many people, adapting to loss involved incorporating some aspect of their previous relationship with the deceased person into their current lives but in a way that was tolerable and not distressing.

Evaluation of social approaches and their application to organ donation contexts

Social approaches to understanding loss highlight that people are situated in particular societies and cultures and have important roles and relationships which transcend what goes on in their minds. Bereavement changes the roles they occupy and the relationships available to them. This is important because many people define their sense of self through their social roles such as being a parent or having a good job. Box 2.3 describes the implications of these models for organ donation situations. The need to talk to other members of the family, to be with the critically ill person and to talk about them to each other and to staff are all explained within a framework of creating a *durable biography* (Walter 1996). These approaches suggest that near the time of death and afterwards, families start to transform their relationship bonds to the critically ill living person and develop a continuing relationship with the deceased person (Klass *et al.* 1996). These models arise out of the living conditions and experiences of developed countries where people tend to have less socially-enmeshed relationships. They also assume that verbal fluency is necessary to create biographies.

Box 2.3 Implications of social approaches for organ donation situations

- They highlight the importance of society and culture in determining reactions to loss and organ donation.
- Structural aspects such as age, gender and social status are recognized as important in constructing social responses to a death.
- As many potential donors are children, these approaches to understanding loss highlight contemporary values placed upon each child by parents in countries where family sizes are small.
- These models highlight the social changes that bereaved people face, such as becoming a widow or a childless mother.
- They suggest that families may need time to engage in the narrative work in constructing the biography of the dying and deceased person. These biographies may also be influential in helping to make donation decisions, for example, by describing the deceased person as someone who would like to help others, and attributing altruism to them.

- The coming together of family members in the hospital to construct the biography may be seen as helpful and supportive.
- It is necessary to recognize the importance of allowing families to tell their story and talk about the critically ill person, often repeatedly. This helps to construct the identity of the ill person when staff may have little knowledge about his or her social roles, attributes and beliefs.
- Some families may gain benefit in deriving a meaning for the death in permitting organ donation, but this should not be assumed for all.
- Some families may wish to obtain mementos of the deceased such as a lock of hair, a photograph or piece of jewellery as a ritual object to help create a lasting sense of presence and a focus for a transformed relationship.

Bereavement support interventions

Here I will briefly introduce different types of supportive interventions that are offered to bereaved people. It is likely that most people affected by organ donation requests will have sufficient resources from within themselves, from their own families, social networks or communities to cope well with their grief. In the UK, most bereavement support is provided by self-help groups, faith groups or other community groups rather than through statutory health and social care organizations. However, in certain circumstances the loss may overwhelm an individual's coping abilities and sources of informal support. In these cases, bereaved people may need access to more formal types of support. The assumptions that underpin most types of bereavement support include:

- it is 'good' to talk;
- emotional expression is helpful within certain defined limits and in certain situations;
- emotional disclosure is therapeutic;
- a linear 'progression' over time from higher levels of distress to lower levels of distress;
- an expectation that grieving will lessen and eventually end.

It is not difficult to see that these assumptions are based on the phase and stage models of bereavement described in this chapter as intra-psychic perspectives. They have gained such widespread acceptance that it is not unusual that immediately after a disaster or where there are multiple deaths, bereavement counsellors are sent to the scene to offer debriefing and counselling.

It may be helpful for transplant services and other hospital-based services to consider carefully the types of support which are needed by the families affected by organ donation, in the immediate period around the donation decision and during donation procedures, and in the subsequent bereavement period. In the context of palliative care services, which may also be applicable here, Payne and Lloyd Williams (2003) have proposed a framework for bereavement support with focuses on three dimensions:

- social support such as lunch groups, drop-in centres, coffee meetings;
- educational support such as information leaflets about managing finance or funerals, books about the experience of grief, talks by experts such as lawyers;
- therapeutic interventions such as counselling, psychotherapy, art or drama therapy.

They argue that services need to be clear about the intentions of the bereavement support activities within the three dimensions. However, while services might be directed to one aim, people may also derive additional benefits. For example, members of a therapeutic group may also experience the meetings as socially supportive. For families facing organ donation decisions, the provision of educational information, both verbal and written, about donation options and procedures is vital and in addition they may require information about sources of bereavement support, practical aspects of registering the death, arranging a funeral and dealing with finances. For some people and families, social support may also be helpful, especially if they are going through the experience alone. During the process of organ donation decision-making, they may value the presence of an independent person such as a bereavement volunteer or spiritual support from a hospital faith worker. Later they may wish to access support groups where they can contact others who have undergone similar experiences (the British Organ Donor Society provides such a function). Some people may find the experience of organ donation deeply troubling and may benefit from referral to a counsellor to explore their feelings and thoughts. A few people who experience complicated bereavement reactions may wish to be referred to therapeutic interventions such as one-to-one grief counselling or a therapeutic group.

How effective are bereavement interventions?

There is an assumption that providing bereavement support is beneficial and that bereavement interventions are therapeutic, but what is the evidence for this? Should bereavement support be provided to all families after organ donation or only those with serious problems in coping with their grief? Kato and Mann (1999) conducted a narrative and meta-analysis of bereavement intervention studies and concluded that most psychotherapeutic interventions were not effective for dealing with depression in bereaved people. In another comprehensive review of the literature, Neimeyer (2001) has demonstrated that bereavement interventions are only helpful for those people with existing problems. He concluded that they were ineffective for people with normal grief experiences. Following an extensive review of the evidence, Schut *et al.* (2001) offer the following summary that:

- primary preventative interventions which were open to all bereaved people showed no evidence of effectiveness;
- secondary preventative interventions that were targeted at bereaved people who were assessed as vulnerable and 'at risk' using standardized measures showed modest effectiveness;
- tertiary preventative interventions for bereaved people with complicated grief showed good outcomes.

They recommended that bereavement interventions should be *targeted* only at those with high risk factors and should be *offered* to those who seek help. This suggests that there is little rationale for transplant services in establishing generic bereavement services for all families affected by organ donation, but they might wish to consider undertaking risk assessment of bereaved people to identify those at most risk of poor bereavement outcomes. There are well-recognized attributes of the person, their environment and the nature of the death, which allow predictions to be made about which people need help (see Relf 2004).

Conclusion

Recognition of the different approaches to conceptualizing bereavement and loss has the potential to contribute to knowledge accumulation in organ donation. It is helpful for people working with families and supporting the process of organ donation to challenge the taken-for-granted assumptions that often pervade bereavement support. This chapter has described three approaches to conceptualizing bereavement. It has presented them in three domains: intra-psychic, interactional and social. This categorization may be a useful heuristic device but it is acknowledged that it does not do justice to the complexity of the theories. In reality, many of these approaches would provide explanations that cover all three domains, but it is the emphasis that varies. Each approach has been assessed for the messages and implications it has for people working in organ donation contexts.

Finally, the chapter concluded with a brief consideration of bereavement support interventions and the evidence for their efficacy, which concludes that most interventions are only worthwhile when people are already experiencing complicated grief reactions. Bereavement is an inevitable part of life and the pain of grief a consequence of forming significant relationships. Health care workers will also face losses in their own lives as well as being exposed to the vicarious grief of families. They too need support and the opportunity to acknowledge their own grief.

References

Bartlett, D. (1998) *Stress*. Buckingham: Open University Press.

Bowlby, J. (1969) *Attachment and Loss, Vol. 1: Attachment*. London: The Hogarth Press.

Bowlby, J. (1973) *Attachment and Loss, Vol. 2: Separation*. London: The Hogarth Press.

Bowlby, J. (1980) *Attachment and Loss, Vol. 3: Loss: Sadness and Depression*. London: The Hogarth Press.

Evans, A. (1994) Anticipatory grief: a theoretical challenge, *Palliative Medicine*, 8(2): 159–65.

Field, D. and Payne, S. (2005) Social aspects of bereavement, *Cancer Nursing Practice*, March supplement, 27–9.

Field, D., Hockey, J. and Small, N. (eds) (1997) *Death, Gender and Ethnicity*. London: Routledge.

Folkman, S. (1997) Positive psychological states and coping with severe stress, *Social Science & Medicine*, 45: 1207–21.

Freud, S. (1917) *Mourning and Melancholia*. London: The Hogarth Press.

Giddens, A. (1976) *New Rules of Sociological Method: A Positive Critique of Interpretive Sociologies*. London: Hutchinson.

Hockey, J., Katz, J. and Small, N. (2001) *Grief, Mourning and Death Ritual*. Buckingham: Open University Press.

Kato, P.M. and Mann, T. (1999) A synthesis of psychological interventions for the bereaved, *Clinical Psychology Review*, 19: 279–96.

Kissane, D.W. and Bloch, S. (2002) *Family Focused Grief Therapy*. Buckingham: Open University Press.

Klass, D., Silverman, P.R. and Nickman, S.L. (1996) *Continuing Bonds*. Philadephia, PA: Taylor & Francis.

Kubler-Ross, E. (1969) *On Death and Dying*. New York: Macmillan.

Lazarus, R.S. and Folkman, S. (1984) *Stress, Appraisal and Coping*. New York: Springer-Verlag.

Lofland, L.H. (1985) The social shaping of emotion: a case of grief, *Symbolic Interaction*, 8(2): 171–90.

Neimeyer, R.A. (2001) *Meaning Reconstruction and the Experience of Loss*. Washington, DC: American Psychological Association.

Nolen-Hoeksema, S. (2001) Ruminative coping and adjustment, in M.S. Stroebe,

R.O. Hansson, W. Stroebe and H. Schut (eds) *Handbook of Bereavement Research: Consequences, Coping, and Care*. Washington, DC: American Psychological Association.

Parkes, C.M. (1971) Psychosocial transitions: a field for study, *Social Science & Medicine*, 5(2): 101–14.

Parkes, C.M. (1972) *Bereavement*. London: Routledge.

Parkes, C.M. (1986) *Bereavement*, 2nd edn. London: Routledge.

Parkes, C.M. (1996) *Bereavement*, 3rd edn. London: Routledge.

Parkes, C.M., Laungani, P. and Young, B. (eds) (1997) *Death and Bereavement Across Cultures*. London: Routledge.

Payne, S. and Lloyd-Williams, M. (2003) Bereavement care, in M. Lloyd-Williams (ed.) *Psychosocial Issues in Palliative Care*. Oxford: Oxford University Press.

Payne, S., Horn, S. and Relf, M. (1999) *Loss and Bereavement*. Buckingham: Open University Press.

Reimers, E. (2001) Bereavement – a social phenomenon? *European Journal of Palliative Care*, 8(6): 242–5.

Relf, M. (2004) Risk assessment and bereavement services, in S. Payne, J. Seymour and C. Ingleton (eds) *Palliative Care Nursing: Principles and Evidence for Practice*. Buckingham: Open University Press.

Richardson, R. (2000) *Death, Dissection and the Destitute*. Chicago: University of Chicago Press.

Riches, G. and Dawson, P. (2000) *An Intimate Loneliness: Supporting Bereaved Parents and Siblings*. Buckingham: Open University Press.

Schut, H., Stroebe, M., van den Bout, J. and Terheggen, M. (2001) The efficacy of bereavement interventions: determining who benefits, in M.S. Stroebe, R.O. Hansson, W. Stroebe and H. Schut (eds) *Handbook of Bereavement Research: Consequences, Coping, and Care*. Washington, DC: American Psychological Association.

Seymour, J.E. (2001) *Critical Moments: Death and Dying in Intensive Care*. Buckingham: Open University Press.

Small, N. (2001) Theories of grief: a critical review, in J. Hockey, J. Katz and N. Small (eds) *Grief, Mourning and Death Ritual*. Buckingham: Open University Press.

Sque, M. and Payne, S.A. (1996) Dissonant loss: the experience of donor relatives, *Social Science & Medicine*, 43(9): 1359–70.

Sque, M., Payne, S. and Macleod Clark, J. (2006) Gift of life or sacrifice? Key discourses to understanding organ donor families' decision-making, *Mortality*, 11(2): 117–32.

Stroebe, M. (1992) Coping with bereavement: a review of the grief work hypothesis, *Omega: Journal of Death and Dying*, 26: 19–42.

Stroebe, M. and Schut, H. (1999) The dual process model of coping with bereavement: rationale and description, *Death Studies*, 23: 197–224.

Stroebe, W. and Schut, H. (2001) Risk factors in bereavement outcome: a methodological and empirical review, in M.S. Stroebe, R.O. Hansson, W. Stroebe and H. Schut (eds) *Handbook of Bereavement Research: Consequences, Coping, and Care*. Washington, DC: American Psychological Association.

Stroebe, M.S., Hansson, R.O., Stroebe, W. and Schut, H. (eds) (2001) *Handbook of Bereavement Research: Consequences, Coping and Care*. Washington, DC: American Psychological Association Press.

Stroebe, M.S., Schut, H. and Stroebe, W. (2005) Grief work, disclosure and counselling: do they help the bereaved? *Clinical Psychology Review*, 25(4): 395–414.

Walter, T. (1996) A new model of grief: bereavement and biography, *Mortality*, 1(1): 1–29.

Walter, T. (1999) *On Bereavement*. Buckingham: Open University Press.

Worden, J.W. (1982) *Grief Counselling and Grief Therapy: A Handbook for the Mental Health Practitioner*. New York: Springer.

Worden, J.W. (1991) *Grief Counselling and Grief Therapy*, 2nd edn. New York: Springer.

Worden, J.W. (2001). *Grief Counselling and Grief Therapy*, 3rd edn. New York: Springer.

Wortman, C.B. and Silver, R.C. (1989) The myths of coping with loss, *Journal of Consulting and Clinical Psychology*, 57(3): 349–57.

3 Gift of life or sacrifice? Key discourses for understanding decision-making by families of organ donors

Magi Sque, Sheila Payne and Jill Macleod Clark

Introduction[1]

Globally there is a critical shortage of donor organs to meet the demands for human organ transplantation. An understanding of what motivates families to agree to donation is therefore essential to maximize organ availability. The 'gift of life' is a popular discourse long associated with pro-donation and transplant activists, its use seemingly directed at heightening public awareness about the perceived benefits of organ donation. However, the potential pressure and obligation implicit within such rhetoric could be detrimental to donor families. It has been suggested that the donation event is better re-presented as a 'sacrifice' as this discourse acknowledges the suffering of the bereaved family and the possible difficulties encountered in their decision-making about organ donation. Drawing on data from three studies that explored the bereavement experiences of donor families, this chapter examines the relative value of 'gift of life' or 'sacrifice' as discourses that contribute to a greater understanding of organ donor families' decision-making. We propose that the compelling nature of 'sacrifice' and the manner in which it impinges on families' decision-making may help to explain the high refusal rates in populations that appear generally aware of the benefits of organ transplantation. Insights into the relative importance of 'gift of life' or 'sacrifice' to families when making decisions could potentially contribute to enhancing families' satisfaction with their decisions, improve support to families and increase the incidence of donation.

Background

In the UK approximately 6919 individuals are on the active organ transplant waiting list (UK Transplant 2006), while 90,712 wait for organs in the USA (Organdonor.gov 2006). Relatives of potential deceased donors remain a critical link in maintaining organ supply, as organ donation is normally discussed with them and their support for, agreement or lack of an objection sought, before donation takes place. However, in the UK relatives' refusal rates are 40 per cent overall, rising to 70 per cent among 'non-white' groups (Barber *et al.* 2006). Refusal rates of 50 per cent nationally are noted in the USA (Organdonor.gov 2006), with African Americans donating half as frequently as 'whites'. Clearly, an understanding of what motivates families to agree to donation, or an insight into how they construe their decision-making experience is essential to increase organ availability.

UK and US researchers have elicited factors predictive of families' ability to agree or decline donation by studying the hospital experiences of families who had donation discussed with them, the demographics of the family, and the demographics and wishes of the potential donor (MORI 1995; Sque and Payne 1996; Franz *et al.* 1997; Burroughs *et al.* 1998; DeJong *et al.* 1998; Siminoff *et al.* 2001; Sque *et al.* 2005; Barber *et al.* 2006). Primarily the most deep-seated and pervasive reason for agreeing or declining donation was knowledge of the deceased's wishes, particularly if their wishes had been discussed with the family, or the family believed they would have agreed or declined donation. Families also shared a number of concerns which included not understanding death certified by neurological criteria, not wanting surgery to the body, fearing that the body would be disfigured, and feeling the deceased had suffered enough.

A number of socio-demographic and service factors have been linked to families' positive donation decisions including 'white' ethnicity, pro-donation beliefs, no family conflict about the decision and satisfaction with the quality of care received by the donor and family in hospital. Additional factors relate to the perception that the donation discussion was timely and that it was carried out by experienced staff members, who could answer the families' questions and give information in such a way as to be reassuring about the donation process.

In comparison, factors associated with families declining donation included 'non-white' ethnicity, divisions within the family about the decision, less satisfaction with the quality of care the deceased and family received in hospital, perceptions that the family was surprised, pressured or harassed about donation decisions, untimely information, individual needs not being addressed, feelings about not coping with the decision and wanting to be present when the ventilator was shut down.

While the predictive factors identified above provide some information about families' donation, decision-making they do not provide deeper-level insights or a potential conceptual framework that could explain what facilitates, harnesses and drives families' decisions. A greater understanding of decision-making mechanisms could potentially impact positively on donation rates. Portmann (1999), for instance, has championed the role of autonomy and guardianship of the body as overriding issues in decision-making about organ donation. While these ideas may indeed help to explain donation decisions, Zutlevics (2002) argues that they reflect a narrow view of families' experiences and decision-making.

Early in the era of organ donation, donation began to be described as an act of giving, encouraging voluntarism and altruism, especially when it became clear that a constant supply of organs would be necessary to meet the growing demand (Gerrand 1994). Gerrand suggests that this occurred by equating the new unfamiliar activity of donation with gift-giving, which is widely practised, familiar and popular. The gift-giving discourse highlighted the ultimate worth of donation, embraced sensitivity to the distress of grief-stricken relatives and preserved the notion that the body is not property that can be owned or traded. However, Siminoff and Chillag (1999) argue that while the 'gift of life' slogan reflects the ethic of voluntarism and altruism on which the entire system of organ donation is predicated and may have been useful in educating the public about organ donation, it has not proved effective in maximizing agreement to the donation of organs. Even in western populations where there is high public awareness about the benefits of organ transplantation (Johnson and Goldstein 2003), refusal rates remain high. The 'gift of life' discourse may therefore be over-simplistic in this context, potentially carrying complex and contradictory meanings that may have unexpected effects on those involved in the 'gift relationship' of donation and transplantation (Tutton 2002). In this regard Holtkamp (2002: xxvi) proposes that the 'uplifting' experience of donation for some may also provoke great anxiety: 'Without hesitation, families report that there is great comfort in knowing that something uplifting and noble came from the hateful death of a loved one. However, an abundance of anecdotal information indicates there is more to the story'. This effect can be detected in the following quote by a mother about her son's donation: 'It is an ache that never goes away! An emptiness that can't be filled. A jigsaw puzzle with now 2 pieces missing! I am incomplete' (Holtkamp 2002: 115).

Recently Mongoven (2003) has developed earlier ideas derived from Fox (1996), arguing that the gift in donating relationships is best understood through religious and secular terms of sacrifice. She suggests that transplant policy which seeks to make donation a commonplace routine may leave the donors and their families invisible with the real costs and benefits of their sacrifice unrecognized. The potential for the discourse of sacrifice to provide insights into donor families' decision processes has yet to be explored.

In this chapter we examine the relevance and importance of the two discourses, the 'gift of life' and 'sacrifice', to families' decision-making about organ donation and discuss how each may affect their motivation and decisions. We start with a critical review of organ donation in relation to 'gift of life' and 'sacrifice' discourses.

Organ donation and the gift relationship

The 'gift of life' discourse enshrines the ethos of organ donation (Vernale and Packard 1990; Siminoff and Chillag 1999; Lauritzen *et al.* 2001; Kuczewski 2002). It is embedded in the rhetoric of the pro-donation lobby and the promotion, philosophy and legislation of a number of powerful organizations. In the USA, for instance, recognition was given to the nature of this non-commercial transfer of organs at both federal and state level in The Uniform Anatomical Gift Act that constitutes the legal requirements for donation (WHO 1991). The Human Tissue Authority set up to implement the British Human Tissue Act of 2004 that overhauled previous laws with regard to the use of human organs and tissues has the 'gift relationship' as one of its guiding principles for the acquisition of organs or tissues from a living or deceased person (Human Tissue Authority 2005). More recently The Council of Europe and the World Health Organization (WHO) endorsed a universal 'gift for life' logo at the launch of the First World Day for Organ Donation and Transplantation held in Geneva on 14 October 2005.

The seminal work of Titmuss (1970) on the gift relationship in health and welfare draws heavily on the ideas of early anthropologists, and particularly of Mauss (1990).[2] Mauss described gift exchange theory, the first systematic study of the custom of exchanging gifts, following comparative research among ancient societies of the American Northwest, the islands of Melanesia and Polynesia. Gift exchange constituted the oldest form of economy, rooted in a largely formal and prescribed system of exchange that had certain significance to the tribes in which it was observed. Gift exchange is embedded in notions of ritual and obligation that may not apply fully to organ donation. Nevertheless, it does offer some insights into the processes of *reciprocity* and *kinship* shown to be important in the donation event (Siminoff and Chillag 1999; Sque 2000).

Mauss argued that gifts were never 'free' and that gift-giving behaviour could be predicted. He suggested that the act of giving a gift is a form of contract governed by three major concepts: *the obligation to give, the obligation to receive* and *the obligation to repay*. The act of giving therefore carries with it an expectation of reciprocity, which, if not fulfilled, can be detrimental to the givers and receivers through *the tyranny of the gift* (Fox 1996), the degree of responsibility and indebtedness that giving and receiving evokes. Mauss also suggested that in giving one shares part of oneself. The gift carries with it part of the giver's nature or spirit that creates a bond between the giver and the receiver. He postulated that this *spirit of the gift* represents an inner, animate force in the object exchanged, invested with life and possessing the individuality of the giver.

However, in applying an over-simplistic discourse to donation as the 'gift of life', it is arguable that the importance of reciprocity is overlooked. Thus, while it may be a good thing to give the gift of an organ to save the life of a needy recipient, the inability of the recipient to reciprocate a gift of equal value (i.e. life itself) has the potential to engender disturbing psychological dissonance for both the donating family and the recipient (Sque and Payne 1994; Siminoff and Chillag 1999; Sque 2000; Sque *et al.* 2003).

Mauss utilized gift exchange ideas to explain social cohesion, loyalty and solidarity in early societies, notions that are confirmed by other writers (Hyde 1983; Douglas 1990). However, while organ donation remains a matter of choice in the modern health care system, the autonomy exerted by individuals in making donation choices, coupled with the anonymous donation to an unknown recipient does not satisfy Mauss' requirement of the socially overt obligations to give, receive and repay. Frow (1996) has also argued that, unlike their purpose in early societies, gifts have no longer any overarching social purpose other than at a purely personal level in today's world. Tutton (2002), however, reinforces the use of the gift analogy by suggesting that the discourse of gift has achieved a certain metaphorical resonance as part of a broader political discourse within health care systems that value social equality, altruism, community and a lack of commercialism, as opposed to an alternative trade in body parts.

It could be argued therefore that the adoption of the 'gift of life' discourse may play its most useful role as a vehicle for transplant propaganda, which is designed to act as a driver for voluntary, altruistic donation based on valuing human life. This ethos counters commercialism and market-based exchanges, and potentially ensures continuance of the transplant programme and all that depends on it.

While organ donation has been widely represented by the discourse as a special and extraordinary gift, this ignores both the context in which the family who must decide about donation find themselves and the issues that impinge on their decision-making. A key question to consider is the extent to which the 'gift of life' discourse provides an understanding of families' behaviour when faced with donation choices. The gift of an organ is precious and comes at a high cost through an often sudden and tragic death and the burden of donation for the family.

Organ donation as sacrifice

Mongoven (2003) has offered an alternative view of the process of organ donation, equating it to a 'sacrifice'. The notion of sacrifice has been handed down through the ages within religious traditions as an offering made valuable by a hard-wrought, difficult-to-relinquish gift or an offering aimed at maintaining connections between humans and their gods (Hubert and Mauss 1964). The act of sacrifice is complex and sacrifices can take many forms. However, the overriding tradition involves the shedding of blood through the slaughter of an animal or human, often severing the neck, slitting the throat, removing the heart or cutting the sacrificed object into pieces. Hubert and Mauss describe sacrifice as having a number of stages involving those who make the sacrifice, the sacrificer, the object of sacrifice and the receiver of the offering. Furthermore, the sacrificer must be prepared to undertake the sacrifice and to be deeply affected by being present at the offering and the role they play in it. Such sacrifices, that affect the sacrificer directly, are termed *personal sacrifices*.

Metaphorically, *personal sacrifices* are used to describe good deeds or signify gifts to other humans that are usually wrought at great individual expense. Mongoven (2003) proposes that organ donation fulfils the criteria of sacrifice. The bereaved family must make the often very difficult decision to relinquish the guardianship and protection of the corpse to allow the cutting up of the body and the removal of organs, albeit through a standardized surgical procedure, for the benefit of the recipient (Sque *et al.* 2003).

Mongoven acknowledges two distinctive and important dimensions of sacrifice; namely the motivational and the cultic dimensions. The motivational aspect reflects the intent of the sacrifice, which in the case of organ donation is giving the 'gift of life'. The cultic aspect reflects the routinized, standardized means of achieving the donation through the certification of death using neurological, brain-based criteria, keeping the body on ventilator support and cutting up of the body and removing the organs at the donation operation.

It is highly likely that the discourses of both 'gift of life' and 'sacrifice' play key roles in the complex family decision-making concerning organ donation. However, there is no empirical data to support this supposition. Similarly little is known about the relative importance and relevance of these discourses to families.

Method

To gain insights into the relevance of 'sacrifice' or the 'gift of life' as discourses that inform families' decision-making about donation and the importance of these discourses, we reviewed data from a series of three studies carried out between 1996–2003 with donor families, searching for evidence of explicit or metaphorical discourses that represented either 'sacrifice' or 'gift of life'.

The first dataset (D1) comprised transcripts of individual, tape-recorded, qualitative, cross-sectional interviews carried out with 24 relatives of 16 organ donors in the UK (Sque and Payne 1996). These data were originally collected to explore relatives' experiences of the donation process. Interviews examined relatives' emotional reactions to the death of a family member and donation of their organs, their perceptions of the decision-making process and the benefits and concerns that organ donation generated for them.

The second dataset (D2) was derived from an investigation carried in four USA organ procurement organizations (OPOs) and the National Donor Family Council (NDFC) (Sque 2000). The OPO dataset, from 333 donors, spanning an eight-year period, comprised 554 letters written by donor families to recipients and 744 letters written by recipients to donor families. The NDFC dataset consisted of 93 letters written to the NDFC by donor families. The study sought to explore the bereavement of donor families by establishing the role and importance of corresponding with transplant recipients and the nature and pattern of the correspondence. Letters were analysed for their pattern of interaction and thematically for content. The present review only accessed letters written by donor families.

The third dataset (D3) was drawn from a three-year, longitudinal study that investigated the bereavement experiences of 47 donor relatives of 41 donors (Sque *et al.* 2003). Relatives were interviewed at three time points: 3–5 months, 13–15 months and 15–26 months post-bereavement. Interview data were analysed using thematic analysis.

Full ethical approval was gained and ethical principles and mechanisms followed for each of the studies.

The studies cover a spectrum of families' experiences through cross-sectional and longitudinal investigations, providing a large sample of data to be explored, drawing on two types of data: interview responses and correspondence. The UK and the USA broadly share similar systems of involving families in decision-making with regard to organ donation. The datasets therefore provided the potential to explore cross-cultural similarities and differences. The limitations of drawing on relatively small, non-representative samples that did not include families who chose not to donate organs are acknowledged. We are also cognizant of the retrospective nature of the data, which could have afforded participants time for reflection, and which could have been influenced by the audience with whom the family was engaged, i.e. a researcher, recipient or the NFDC.

The three datasets were interrogated for evidence of families' literal, symbolic or metaphorical representations of 'sacrifice' or 'gift of life' discourses in describing their experiences of donation. Representations of 'sacrifice' or the 'gift of life' were grouped under the three broad themes of *'motivation to donate'*, *'letting go'* and *'perceptions of the donation operation'*.

Evidence of literal, symbolic or metaphorical representations related to the discourses of 'gift of life' or 'sacrifice' are presented as exemplar quotes from transcripts, identified by codes. Data from D1 are identified with a code starting with 1 followed by the interview code, while identifiers for D2 data start with 2 and D3 data with 3.

Findings

Many examples were found within the datasets to support the argument that both 'gift of life' and 'sacrifice' discourses are potentially relevant to donor families' decision-making. These exemplars support the notion that the 'gift of life' discourse is strongly linked to *'motivation to donate'*. The discourse of 'sacrifice' was also evident in participants' decision-making process and the emotional context of donation, particular in the themes of *'letting go'* and *'perceptions of the donation operation'*.

The gift of life

Motivation to donate

Clear examples of the centrality of 'the gift of life' to families' motivation to donate can be seen in the following quotes.

A wife whose husband died on Christmas Eve said:

What a lovely Christmas present to save somebody's life. (1.15)

A father who was talking about his son's donation:

It's not a reward that you get, it's something that happens as a result of a loved one wishing to give their organs to somebody else. They give their organs to somebody else so that they can have the gift of life and what they give to us is almost not an easy road in grief but a different road through grief, a less harsh road, and a less final death, because it is a death filled with different emotions, it's filled with the joy of knowing good has come out of his death, as opposed to us having to know that, just, ah, nothing has come out of his death, only pain and sorrow and sadness and also knowing that it is not only the recipient that receives, it's their family, their friends ... It is a tremendous thing, it ripples out to hundreds of people ... Almost unending the relief and saving of pain that just giving something that is not needed can produce. (1.16)

Donor parents writing to the NDFC:

It is also wonderful to know that because of my son there are three people in the world who have a new chance of life and at the same time, two also have new sight because of T, so a wonderful part of T *still lives* on and we are so proud of him. (2.NF 17)

On a sad day a couple of months later, the letter arrived telling us about the recipients of J's organs, corneas and tissues. My tears were now mixed with gratitude. Our generous, outgoing, caring son will live in others. What a precious gift for all. (2.NF 45)

And then he [recipient] told us how thankful he was to receive a new heart. He was living a life to take special care of it with no smoking, no drinking, good diet and exercise. He was living a productive life for the first time in many years. He was working and giving thanks every day for 'the gift that gave him a second chance of life'. We felt so blessed to know that our child's heart was giving a new life to this man and his family. (2.NF 82)

A donor mother writing to the NDFC about the gift of sight her son gave through his death reported:

Somewhere along the way, D discovered what policemen were, what they did and that his dad was one of them. He thought that cops were the greatest people on earth. D grew up with the police department, spending countless hours with cops watching them, talking to them, admiring them and dreaming about one day becoming a police   officer himself. But D never realized that the very disabilities [spina bifida] that made him so special would also keep him from being the cop he had always wanted to be ... In his death D was able to save the sight and career of a police officer. And in so doing he became the cop he had always wanted to be. (2.NF 74)

Donor parents writing to the recipient of their son's organs:

> We are glad to hear that you [recipient] are doing well and it is good to know that the heart of our very special, very well loved little boy is still giving life to someone. (2.DV 105)

Although organ donation is not obligatory, it has been suggested that there are subtle social pressures that enhance *the obligation to give*. Media coverage has also increased the public's awareness of the need for donor organs by highlighting the purposeful nature of transplantation, often through well-known public figures who have received a transplant. In other instances, highly publicized persons, waiting for organs, have become household names. The emotive nature of these stories creates their own subversive pressures on families that may become involved in the donation process. Religious traditions also value the conviction that to give to others is supremely good. The consequences of such gift-giving are assumed to be beneficial to the donor, the recipient and the wider society (Vernale and Packard 1990). It is possible that for a time the essential bonds of kinship common in early societies are rekindled (even if complete anonymity between donor and recipient is maintained) in an ultimate concern for another person. From this viewpoint, the more widespread the personal and collective commitment to the concept of a gift that makes us our stranger's keeper, as well as our brother's keeper, the more ideal society is supposed to be (Titmuss 1970).

The sacrifice

Letting go

Families appeared, at great emotional cost to themselves, reluctant to 'let go' and relinquish their guardianship and ability to protect the body, even if it meant offering a lifeline to recipients. The cultic dimension of sacrifice in deceased donation demands the removal of organs from a donor who although certified dead by neurological criteria, is maintained on a ventilator and may not look dead. This makes the imagery of a living sacrifice even more acute. Here a wife describes her difficulty in saying goodbye to her recently deceased husband before leaving him.

I: How did you actually make that decision to go and say goodbye?

P: Well, it is very difficult to. All I kept thinking was that, I kept saying to my brother-in-law, 'How can you say goodbye to somebody who is still breathing?' I mean, Oh God, I kept on saying, 'He's warm, he's still perspiring, he's warm.' Because to me he wasn't dead really . . . because he was still breathing. And I know it was the machine and that, but he was too warm. How can you say goodbye to somebody that is? (1.05)

Here a father describes his experience of 'letting go' his son, which he later described as the worst experience of his life.

It is very difficult to make that definite decision and say we are prepared for you to take A into a theatre and remove the very vital organs that would enable him to live. So that meant that we, needed to be sure, or I needed to be sure, a 100 per cent, that there was no chance for A to sustain life for himself and that was why I asked to be at the final brainstem test . . . then doubting what I had seen I thought, well, perhaps, I'll see some hope if I look up, and I looked up at the others standing round the bed and they were all crying, everyone of them, and I just knew that these weren't nurses and doctors, these were just ordinary people, these were mums and dads, just ordinary people, like we were, and if they could have done anything they would have done it, there was no way they were going to put themselves through this sort of anguish if they could have avoided it, and so it absolutely underlined for me that if there was anything at all that could have been done to help him it would have been done. (1.16)

Richardson (2000) found that the protection of the physical body is a recurring characteristic of popular death customs. The cadaver is no longer the person; nonetheless, the expectation is that even after death the body is treated with care, respect and ritual reverence for the sake of the person whom it represented. Families in these examples were clearly concerned about the treatment of the deceased and sought to continue to protect them. A father reports how he could not allow donation of his daughter's corneas:

She looked so beautiful, she wasn't marked in anyway, can't cut these eyes out you know, that's how I sort of visualized it then. (1.12)

He was concerned about her vulnerability at the donation operation:

I wanted to protect her more, because I mean, she was very vulner-able, wasn't she? For all intents and purposes she was dead, but I did not want her to be cut about. I didn't want her to be injured. You see she was not injured in my eyes, because there were no marks. So anything done after that would be an operation, and I couldn't comprehend that too much, at that particular time. So really that was my reservation, I didn't want her to be hurt. (1.12)

Perceptions of the donation operation

Participants used graphic imagery in relation to their perceptions of the donation operation. They appeared concerned about the mutilation, 'cultic' part of sacrifice acted out through the donation operation and the perceived prolonged suffering of the donor. A father perceives the prolonged suffering of his daughter:

> Concerned about the tragic way she was taken from us and was it right to do this [donation], she is going through a traumatic death, having gone through such a horrendous death [donation]. (1.09)

A wife talked about her husband and the impact of his perceived suffering on their children:

> You hear horrific stories like, and I think they were a bit worried they might slit him open and, and put a sticky plaster over him and patch him up again, I mean we don't know what goes on and he had been through so much, that I think one of A's problems and T's [children] may be was that they did not want him to suffer any more. Yeah, to us he was on the ventilator, his chest was still going up and down and yet they wanted to cut him open and take all his bits and pieces away before he'd even, well, you know, to us he wasn't dead because he was, we could still see. I know it was a ventilator, we know that, but to us he was still breathing because the machine was still going up and down, and to us he was still alive and yet they wanted to go and cut him open and dig all his bits ... It was just so hard to accept for me and T that that's what they wanted to do. (1.11)

A mother visualized the donation operation:

> I just had these horrible visions of you know, of sort of, you know, like a piece of meat you know, stuck, dash and get it out and be done with. Like I say my visions was messy and all slapdash business. (1.08)

A father articulated his thoughts about the donation operation:

> I thought G was going to be carved up. (1.09)

As do the following participants who were talking about their deceased wives:

I've got my wife dying and I've got people want to cut her open and rip bits out of her. (3.32483,32568)

Someone would go in there and just be tearing her to bits I couldn't have that. (3.58632,58711)

All you know is that they are going to rip her open and I was concerned. (3.44772,44843)

Sacrifice or the gift of life: A dilemma for the donor family?

Data from the three studies revealed many examples of descriptions by participants which can be linked to 'gift of life' discourse. Similarly several explicit or metaphorical examples were also found which were related to cutting, and mutilation, relevant to the cultic notion of sacrifice. These examples evidenced the nature of hard-wrought decision-making for families and the existence of their emotional and physical sacrifice. Examples drawn from these three datasets not only support donor families' perceptions of the decision-making process but serve to illuminate potential explanations for families who decline donation.

The 'gift of life' motivation for donation appeared to be very important to some families and it is interesting to note that families employed the 'gift of life' and 'gift of sight' discourse as well as referring to the actual giving of an organ, such as the heart. This suggests the view that, to families, the donation had a greater value than a mere physical object or tissue, agreeing with Mauss' (1990) concept of *the spirit of the gift*. Moloney and Walker (2002) concur with Mongoven (2003) suggesting that the 'gift of life' discourse is linked to perceptions of life, rather than the death of the donor and the suffering of the bereaved family. If this is the case then within the 'gift of life' context the families' roles could be relegated to the mere provision of spare parts.

From data reported here it is notable that while families embraced the notion of 'gift of life' as a worthy outcome of donation they also appeared to be struggling with the biomedical and cultic, sacrificial requirements of the donation process. This raises questions about the ethics of promoting 'the gift of life' discourse. Media representation does not take account of the suffering that organ donation and transplantation causes through *the tyranny of the gift* (Fox 1996). The powerful influences that a donated or transplanted organ can exert over the lives of those concerned are sources of this tyranny. This struggle has been highlighted by other authors (MORI 1995; Sque and Payne

1996; Franz *et al.* 1997; Burroughs *et al.* 1998; DeJong *et al.* 1998; Siminoff *et al.* 2001; Sque *et al.* 2005; Barber *et al.* 2006). Family members in the examples reported here clearly made their decisions against a backdrop of not wanting the body to be cut, fear that the body would be disfigured and the thought that the deceased had suffered enough.

Interrogation of the data also revealed the difficulties experienced by families in 'letting go' of the deceased and handing over guardianship of the body to allow the donation operation to take place. Even with knowledge of its decay Richardson (2000) argues that the corpse's position has been counterpoised by a profound conception of metaphysical attributes such as sentience, spiritual power, transitory existence and an afterlife. A corpse can inspire solicitude and sentimentality, as well as fear; even when the living individual may never have done so. Portmann (1999: 228) suggests that an underlying commitment to the preservation of the integrity of the corpse conflicts with the respect for life that can be given through the transplanta-tion of organs: 'We want to guard vigilantly the boundary our bodies created against others and at the same time to open the boundary to others'. These societal pressures may create a dilemma and confusion for families faced with a donation decision. We propose therefore that the notion of sacrifice is compelling. The manner in which sacrifice impinges on families' decision-making, is borne out in the difficulties donor families expressed about their decision-making related to 'letting go' and their 'perceptions of the donation operation', contribute to the *tyranny of the gift*. These perspectives may help to explain that while there is high awareness of the benefits of organ donation and transplantation in the public domain, in many countries refusal rates remain high at the bedside (Barber *et al.* 2006).

Donor families experience an unusual encounter both with death, which is certified by neurological criteria, and with potentially difficult decisions about donation. From the data interrogated here it appears that they identify at least two pervasive discourses about donation as 'gift of life' or 'sacrifice' and the choices to honour their deceased relative. It is possible that the dis-course of 'sacrifice' assumes a greater than hitherto recognized significance for the family at the bedside, faced with a donation decision. Mongoven (2003) cautions that to make organ donation a commonplace routine or any attempt to ritualize donation policy renders the donor's and the family's sacrifice invisible and deflects attention from the real costs and benefits of their sa-crifice. If this is indeed the case then successful donation discussions with families need to be underpinned with an appreciation of the tension that exists between their concerns about their 'sacrifice' and the motivation to give the 'gift of life'. The success of such discussions will be judged not in terms of a positive donation decision but a decision with which the family remains satisfied over time, whatever their decision about donation.

A deeper understanding of how the 'gift of life' and 'sacrifice' discourses compete at the bedside, and the tension that exists between them, is required to provide information which health professionals can use to guide interaction with families on a more informed basis. This has particular implications for the nature and context of information transmitted to donor families about the precise nature of the donation operation.

The complexity of unexpected death and the multiple new experiences associated with the act and process of organ donation make the initiation of discussion about donation and obtaining the agreement of relatives problematic. Approaching a grieving family about organ donation is believed to be one of the most emotionally draining experiences in health care practice (Stoeckle 1990; Featherstone 1994). Childress (2001) suggested that excessively rationalistic donation policies that neglect deep beliefs, symbols, sentiments and emotions attributed to the human body and its parts can become barriers to donation. Maloney and Altmaier (2003) also report findings that show that trained donation professionals report greater confidence in their ability to perform procedural tasks associated with the donation discussion than in their ability to manage affective or emotion-laden issues related to the process. These recent findings suggest that donation professionals appear to continue to have difficulty in raising the question of donation with families, show a lack of understanding about families' decision-making process and their true motivations for donating, as well as about how the experience of being a donor family member affects conversation. These and other reasons could contribute to the disappointing donation consent rates in many countries.

There has been an evolution of expert educational initiatives for donation professionals, such as the European Donor Hospital Education Programme (Cohen and Wight 1999), which aims to improve professionals' understanding of the legal and ethical issues involved in transplantation, help them communicate effectively and sympathetically with bereaved families, and increase organ donation rates. The Donor Action Programme was set up by professional organizations in the USA and Europe to, among other things, sensitize health professionals as to how the needs of bereaved families can be met in a caring and sensitive manner (Cohen and Wight 1999). Spain, the country that leads the world in organ donation and transplantation rates, and the only country where renal transplant waiting lists have decreased every year since 1991, is widely recognized to have achieved this success through, among other things, specifically trained, enthusiastic donation professionals (Martinez *et al.* 2001; Matesanz and Miranda 2002). It is therefore vital to explore any strategies or interventions that have the potential to positively influence donation rates and leave families satisfied with their decision.

Further research designed to enhance understanding of the complex processes underpinning donation decision-making is urgently needed. In particular there is a need to explore the importance of the 'gift of life' and 'sacrifice' discourses in the decision-making process. Such research should include those families who choose not to donate as well as those who do. The extent to which timing of information may influence whether the positive sense of the donation process as a 'gift of life' is more powerful than the potentially negative construct of 'sacrifice' also requires examination.

Conclusion

This chapter provides some unique insights into the complex process of organ donation, through the examination of the discourses related to 'gift of life' and 'sacrifice'. While for some families the decision to offer the 'gift of life' was highly motivating, the decision-making process for others appeared to be linked to deep-seated concerns about the sacrificial element of this gift-giving. The decisions were made in the context of deeply distressing concerns, which could be related to the cultic criteria of sacrifice. Continuing to articulate organ donation within a 'gift of life' discourse remains over-simplistic as it does not reflect the depth and complexity of the process. A decision to facilitate the removal of the vital organs of the deceased, who does not look dead, through post-mortem surgical intervention upon the body, should never be underestimated.

Although the 'gift of life' discourse may remain useful for heightening public awareness about the benefits of donation, this is not an adequate framework for understanding what is important for the family at the bedside faced with a donation decision. We argue that such decisions are more closely related to sacrifice. If this is indeed the case, it provides a potentially valuable framework for explaining the decisions of families who choose not to donate. It may also have some value in explaining why in populations where there is high awareness of donation, refusal rates also remain high. Most importantly it could provide a more supportive framework for guiding future interactions between health care professionals and potential donor families.

Acknowledgements

The authors wish to thank Midwest Organ Bank Inc., Nebraska Organ Retrieval System Inc., LifeGift Organ Donation Center, Gift of Life Donor Program and the National Donor Family Council for facilitating the research carried out in Dataset 2.

Notes

1 Original publication Sque, M., Payne, S. and Macleod, J. (2006) Gift of life or sacrifice? Key discourses to understanding organ donor families' decision-making, *Mortality*, 11(2): 117–32.
2 1990 English translation by Halls W.D. of Mauss' *Essai sur le don* (The gift), first published in 1950 in *Sociologie et Anthropologie* by Presses Universitaires de France.

References

Barber, K., Falvey, S., Hamilton, C., Collett, D. and Rudge, C. (2006) Potential for organ donation in the United Kingdom: audit of intensive care records, *British Medical Journal*, 332: 1124–7.

Burroughs, T.E., Hong, B.A., Kappel, D.F. and Freedman, B.K. (1998) The stability of family decisions to consent or refuse organ donation. Would you do it again? *Psychosomatic Medicine*, 60: 156–62.

Childress, J. F. (2001) The failure to give: reducing barriers to organ donation, *Kennedy Institute of Ethics Journal*, 11: 1–16.

Cohen, B. and Wight, C. (1999) A European perspective on organ procurement: breaking down barriers to organ donation, *Transplantation*, 68: 985–90.

DeJong, W., Franz, H.G., Wolfe, S.M., Nathan, H., Payne, D., Reitsma, W. and Beasley, C. (1998) Requesting organ donation: an interview study of donor and non-donor families, *American Journal of Critical Care*, 7: 13–23.

Douglas, M. (1990) No free gifts. Foreword to *The Gift, the Form and Reason for Exchange in Archaic Societies*. London: Routledge.

Featherstone, K. (1994) Nurses' knowledge and attitudes toward organ and tissue donation in a community hospital, *Journal of Trauma Nursing*, 1: 57–63.

Fox, R.C. (1996) Afterthoughts: continuing reflections on organ transplantation, in S.J. Youngner, R.C. Fox, and L.J. O'Connell (eds) *Organ Transplantation: Meanings and Realities*. Madison, WI: University of Wisconsin Press.

Franz, H.G., DeJong, W., Wolfe, S,M., Nathan, H., Payne, D., Reitsma, W. and Beasley, C. (1997) Explaining brain death: a critical feature of the donation process, *Journal of Transplant Coordination*, 7: 14–21.

Frow, J. (1996) Information as gift and commodity, *New Left Review*, 219: 89–108.

Gerrand, G. (1994) The notion of gift-giving and organ donation, *Bioethics*, 8: 127–50.

Holtkamp, S. (2002) *Wrapped in Mourning: The Gift of Life and Organ Donor Family Trauma*. New York: Brunner-Routledge.

Hubert, H. and Mauss, M. (1964) *Sacrifice: Its Nature and Function*. London: Cohen & West.

Human Tissue Act (2004) London: HMSO.

Human Tissue Authority (2005) *Human Tissue Authority: Draft Codes of Practice for Consultation*. London: Human Tissue Authority.

Hyde, L. (1983) *The Gift, Imagination and the Erotic Life of Property*. New York: Vintage Books.

Johnson, E. J. and Goldstein, D. (2003) Do defaults save lives? *Science*, 302: 1338–9.

Kuczewski, M. G. (2002) The gift of life and starfish on the beach: the ethics of organ procurement, *The American Journal of Bioethics*, 2: 53–6.

Lauritzen, P., McClure, M., Smith, M.L. and Trew, A. (2001) The gift of life and the common good: the need for a communal approach to organ procurement, *Hastings Center Report*, January–February, 29–35.

Maloney, R. and Altmaier, E.M. (2003) Caring for bereaved families: self-efficacy in the donation request process, *Journal of Clinical Psychology in Medical Settings*, 10: 251–8.

Martinez, J.M., Lopez, J.S., Martin, A., Martin, M.J., Scandroglio, B. and Martin, J.M. (2001) Organ donation and family decision-making within the Spanish system, *Social Science & Medicine*, 53: 405–21.

Matesanz, R. and Miranda, B. (2002) A decade of continuous improvement in cadaveric organ donation: the Spanish model, *Journal of Nephrology*, 15: 22–8.

Mauss, M. (1990) *The Gift, the Form and Reason for Exchange in Archaic Societies*. London: Routledge.

Moloney, G. and Walker, I. (2002) Talking about transplants: social representations and the dialectical, dilemmatic nature of organ donation and transplantation, *British Journal of Social Psychology*, 41: 299–320.

Mongoven, A. (2003) Sharing our body and blood: organ donation and feminist critiques of sacrifice, *Journal of Medicine and Philosophy*, 28: 89–114.

MORI Health Research Unit (1995) *Report of a Two Year Study into Reasons for Relatives' Refusal of Organ Donation*. London: Department of Health.

Organ Donation (2006) www.molbio.princeton.edu/courses/mb427/2001/projects/01/donation.htm (accessed 6 January 2006).

Organdonor.gov. (2006) www.organdonor.gov/about.html The official US government website for organ and tissue donation and transplantation maintained by the Health Resources and Services Administration (HRSA), Healthcare Systems Bureau (HSB) and Division of Transplantation, an agency of the US Department of Health and Human Services (HHS) (accessed 6 January 2006).

Portmann, J. (1999) Cutting bodies to harvest organs, *Cambridge Quarterly of Healthcare Ethics*, 8: 288–98.

Richardson, R. (2000) *Death Dissection and the Destitute*. Chicago: University of Chicago Press.

Siminoff, L.A. and Chillag, K. (1999) The fallacy of the 'gift of life', *Hastings Center Report*, 29: 34–41.

Siminoff, L.A., Gordon, N., Hewlett, J. and Arnold, R.M. (2001) Factors influencing families' consent for donation of solid organs for transplantation, *Journal of the American Medical Association*, 286: 71–7.

Sque, M. (2000) *'A Story to Tell': Post Bereavement Correspondence Between Organ Donor Families, Recipients, Their OPOs and the National Donor Family Council – An American Investigation*. A report of a study funded by The General Nursing Council for England & Wales Trust. University of Surrey, Guildford: UK.

Sque, M. and Payne, S. (1994) Gift exchange theory: a critique in relation to organ transplantation, *Journal of Advanced Nursing*, 19: 45–51.

Sque, M. and Payne, S. (1996) Dissonant loss: the experiences of donor relatives, *Social Science & Medicine*, 43: 1359–70.

Sque, M., Long, T. and Payne, S. (2003) *Organ and Tissue Donation: Exploring the Needs of Families*. Final report of a three-year study commissioned by the British Organ Donor Society, funded by the Community Fund. University of Southampton, Southampton: UK.

Sque, M., Long, T. and Payne, S. (2005) Organ donation: key factors influencing families' decision-making, *Transplantation Proceedings*, 37: 543–6.

Stoeckle, M. (1990) Attitudes of critical care nurses toward organ donation, *Dimensions of Critical Care Nursing*, 9: 354–61.

Titmuss, R.M. (1970) *The Gift Relationship from Human Blood to Social Policy*. London: George Allen & Unwin.

Tutton, R. (2002) Gift relationships in genetics research, *Science as Culture*, 11: 523–42.

UK Transplant (2006) Weekly statistics, www.uktransplant.org.uk/ukt/statistics/latest_statistics/latest_statistics.jsp(accessed 29 July 2006).

Vernale, C. and Packard, S. (1990) Organ donation as gift exchange, *Image Journal of Nursing Scholarship*, 22(4): 239–42.

WHO (1991) *Human Organ Transplantation: A Report on Developments Under the Auspices of WHO*. Geneva: WHO.

Zutlevics, T.L. (2002) Response to 'Cutting Bodies to Harvest Organs' by John Portmann (CQ Vol 8, No 3) Autonomy as scapegoat in the organ shortage debate: a reply to Portmann, *Cambridge Quarterly of Healthcare Ethics*, 11: 68–72.

4 A dissonant loss: the bereavement of organ donor families

Magi Sque

Introduction

Organ and tissue donation usually arises out of situations of acute injury or the onset of severe illness that terminates in the unexpected, sudden death of a relatively young, previously healthy individual. Most studies have focused on provision for specific needs of the bereaved family rather than attempted to capture and describe the nature and meaning of having a relative in a critical care situation that ended in organ donation. Without an adequate understanding of the psychological and social context in which these events unfold, an informative picture cannot be adequately developed about relatives' experience: of what happened, its nature and quality, and how family care may be safeguarded and maximized. Therefore a shift is needed towards an approach that better captures the role of personal meanings, and the complexity and uniqueness of the experience, to understand how families perceived their situation and coped with their often profoundly poignant and rueful circumstances.

Theory derived inductively from research data has the power to explain real-life situations. Revealing the main bereavement concerns of organ donor families through theory derived from their experiences illuminates variables that provide insights to promote best practice. This may be through the ability to predict clinical situations and therefore offer evidence to health care professionals to appropriately support and guide families in their decision-making and bereavement.

This chapter is based on an English study carried out through face-to-face interviews that examined the experiences of relatives of multi-organ donors. Grounded theory (Glaser and Strauss 1967) was used to develop an understanding of relatives' experiences of organ donation. This approach facilitated the development of a theory that could be applied to family care, based on the actual experiences of the individuals involved. Donor relatives' experiences were found to revolve around a theme of conflict and resolution. Their experience was explained as a theory of 'dissonant loss' (Sque 1996; Sque and Payne 1996). The following sections will describe the development of the theory, its implications for practice, and finally offer a critique of the theory.

The theory of dissonant loss

Letters facilitated by transplant coordinators from three regional transplant coordinating services in England invited a purposive sample of relatives from 42 families of organ donors, who had been certified dead using neurological criteria, to join the study. Relatives were chosen for their perceived wide range of experiences of organ donation, such as their relationship to the donor, and geographical location, which could have affected local practices and availability of bereavement support. Twenty-four relatives of 16 organ donors were recruited into the study. Six families declined, 3 were overseas, and 17 did not reply. Table 4.1 provides details of the sample.

All participating next of kin had agreed to multi-organ donation. Twelve donations were requested and four were offered spontaneously. The median age of donors was 26 years, the age range being 10 weeks to 56 years. Donors spent a median of four days in hospital, the range being 1–21 days. Audio-taped, narrative interviews, carried out in participants' homes, gave them the opportunity to talk freely about their experiences.

The study examined relatives' emotional reactions to death and dona-tion, perceptions of the decision-making process, assessment of the problems donation caused for them, as well as the benefits it provided. An under-standing of what the experience meant to them was elicited, as well as identification of their needs. Analysis of interview transcripts was guided by a grounded theory approach, based on the constant comparative method (Glaser and Strauss 1967). A clustering of concepts were classified into themes that were used to form 11 definitive categories. The categories were arranged around the central purpose of the research, *donor relatives' experiences*, to form an analytical version of their story. The model in Figure 4.1 shows the con-ceptual representation of this story.

The model indicates a sequential relationship of 11 identified categories that conceptualized phases of families' donation experiences. These were:

- *'the last time we were together'* – the last occasion the deceased relative and family member were together;
- *finding out something is wrong* – when the family member witnessed the onset of the critical injury or illness or first found out something had happened to their relative;
- *waiting for a diagnosis* – when the family member was waiting for the diagnosis of the critical injury;

Table 4.1 Participant sample to show relationship to donor, donor age, critical injury and time of interview since donation

Relationship to donor	Donor age (years)	Critical injury	Time of interview since donation (months)
Parents	27	Cerebral haemorrhage	5
Parents	25	Cerebral anoxia following cardiopulmonary arrest	7
Parents	20	Head injury following a riding accident	36
Parents	22	Head injury following road traffic accident	8
Parents	26	Marphan's syndrome	18
Parents	10	Viral meningitis	16
Mother	22	Cerebral anoxia following an asthma attack	11
Mother	0*	Cerebral anoxia following asphyxiation	11
Father	26	Head injury following road traffic accident	4
Husband	44	Cerebral haemorrhage	7
Husband	56	Cerebral haemorrhage	8
Husband	48	Cerebral haemorrhage	17
Wife	47	Cerebral haemorrhage	4
Wife	47	Cerebral haemorrhage	18
Wife & mother	22	Head injury following road traffic accident	7
Wife & daughter-in-law	50	Cerebral haemorrhage	4

*baby 10 weeks old

Reprinted from *Social Science & Medicine*, 49(3): Sque, M. and Payne, S., Dissonant loss: the experiences of donor relatives, 1359–70 (1996) with permission from Elsevier.

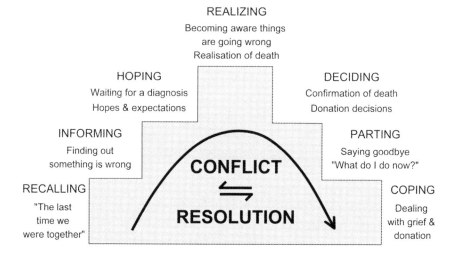

Figure 4.1 A model of donor relatives' experiences

Adapted from *Social Science & Medicine*, 49(3): Sque, M. and Payne, S., Dissonant loss: the experiences of donor relatives, 1359–70 (1996) with permission from Elsevier.

- *hopes and expectations* – hoping that the injured relative would not die and expecting that they would recover;
- *becoming aware that things are going wrong* – the family member becoming aware that recovery of the injured relative is no longer possible;
- *realization of death* – the family member realizes, for themselves, that their relative has died;
- *confirmation of death* – death is confirmed by brainstem testing;
- *donation decisions* – the family member makes decisions about organ donation;
- *saying goodbye* – the family member says goodbye to the deceased relative;
- *'What do I do now?'* – how the family member feels about leaving the intensive care unit;
- *dealing with grief and donation* – how the family member copes with their grief and the outcomes of the donation.

There appeared to be particular behaviours through which participants acted out these phases of their experience. These were:

- *recalling* – when the family member talked about the attributes of their relative and the last occasion they shared together;

- *informing* – when they were first told about or witnessed the onset on their relative's critical injury or illness;
- *hoping* – for recovery during the hospital experience;
- *realizing* – that their relative would not recover;
- *deciding* – about donation;
- *parting* – leaving the relative;
- *coping* – with grief and donation.

These behaviours, which appeared to contribute to participants' ability to move through each phase of the donation process were accompanied by a series of fluctuating and conflicting cognitive and psychological processes, before resolutions to each new situation was accomplished. Participants' behaviours were therefore explained through a process of conflict and resolution that pervaded the categories and formed the core (category) of their experiences. Conflict is defined in this sense as: *'The simultaneously opposing tendencies within the individual or environment, which cause discrepancy, discord, or dissonance, and the distress resulting from these instances'*.

With the identification of the integrating core category, of conflict and resolution, it became possible to focus on how this process was related to each phase of participants' experience and how it was described in accounts of their behaviour. The theory of dissonant loss was therefore developed using the core category of conflict and resolution to explain participants' psychosocial concerns and behaviours during the donation experience. The theory also describes factors that created resolutions to participants' conflicts and helped them move through the phases of the donation process. Dissonant loss is defined as: *'A bereavement or loss, which is characterized by a sense of uncertainty and psychological inconsistency'*.

The loss of the deceased relative was assured but the effects of the loss were surrounded by ambiguity and incompatibility with the participants' familiar world. Dissonance occurred as the loss was encompassed by a series of complex decisions. These decisions were made necessary by the pervasive elements of conflict and resolution. Figure 4.2[1] offers a schematic representation of the theory of dissonant loss and the sources of conflict and resolution experienced by participants.

Conflict and resolution in the donation process: the social context and practice implications

Conflict originated in the short and intensely emotional period of hospitalization. During this time participants appeared to lose control to the professionals, as they were functioning outside of their familiar world. The degree of conflict and dissonance experienced by participants was

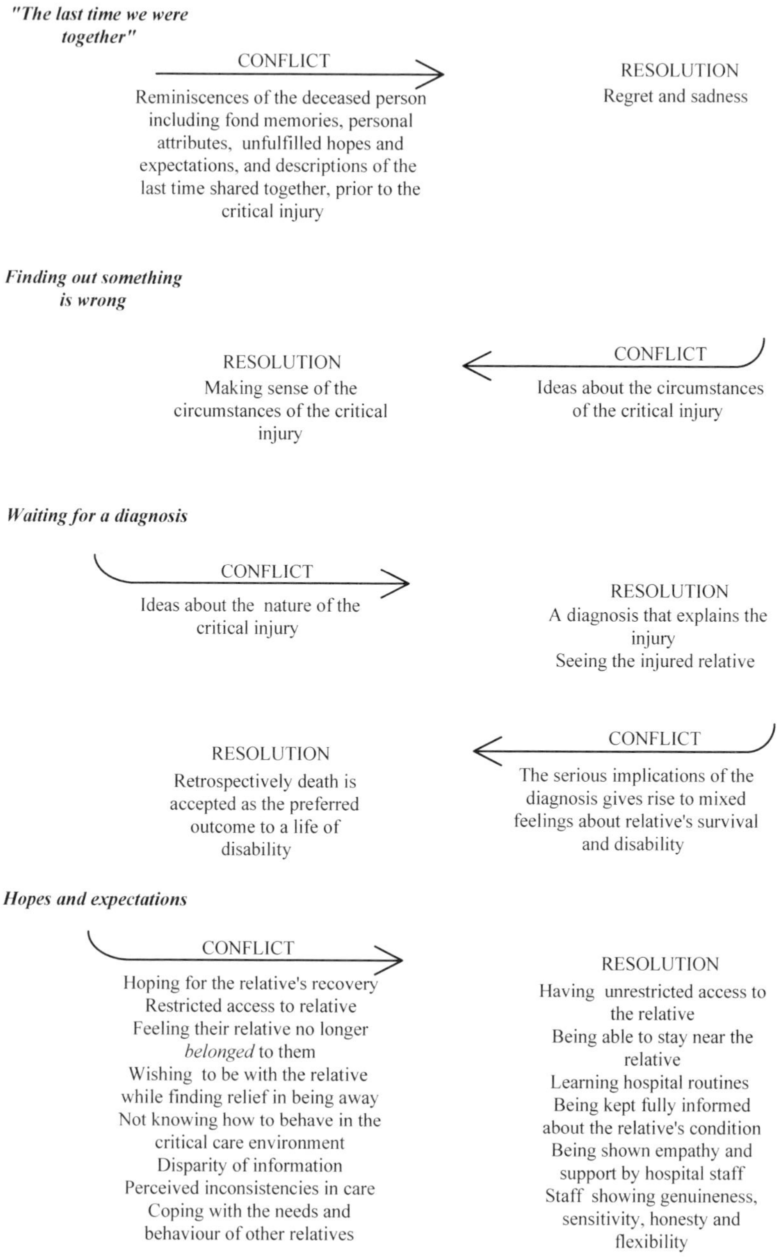

"The last time we were together"

CONFLICT

Reminiscences of the deceased person including fond memories, personal attributes, unfulfilled hopes and expectations, and descriptions of the last time shared together, prior to the critical injury

RESOLUTION

Regret and sadness

Finding out something is wrong

RESOLUTION

Making sense of the circumstances of the critical injury

CONFLICT

Ideas about the circumstances of the critical injury

Waiting for a diagnosis

CONFLICT

Ideas about the nature of the critical injury

RESOLUTION

A diagnosis that explains the injury
Seeing the injured relative

RESOLUTION

Retrospectively death is accepted as the preferred outcome to a life of disability

CONFLICT

The serious implications of the diagnosis gives rise to mixed feelings about relative's survival and disability

Hopes and expectations

CONFLICT

Hoping for the relative's recovery
Restricted access to relative
Feeling their relative no longer *belonged* to them
Wishing to be with the relative while finding relief in being away
Not knowing how to behave in the critical care environment
Disparity of information
Perceived inconsistencies in care
Coping with the needs and behaviour of other relatives

RESOLUTION

Having unrestricted access to the relative
Being able to stay near the relative
Learning hospital routines
Being kept fully informed about the relative's condition
Being shown empathy and support by hospital staff
Staff showing genuineness, sensitivity, honesty and flexibility

Figure 4.2 A theory of dissonant loss

Reprinted from *Social Science & Medicine*, 49(3): Sque, M. and Payne, S., Dissonant loss: the experiences of donor relatives, 1359–70 (1996) with permission from Elsevier.

Becoming aware that
things are going wrong
Realization of death

CONFLICT

Knowing recovery is no
longer possible
Personal realization
of death
Not knowing how to behave
Waiting for confirmation
of death

RESOLUTION
Confirmation of death

Confirmation of Death

RESOLUTION
Confidence in BST
Not seeing the relative once
death is confirmed
Post retrieval viewing of the
body

CONFLICT

Difficult to equate death
with the appearance of
the ventilated relative
Lack of knowledge about
death certified by BST

Donation decisions

CONFLICT

Decisions to be made
about donation

RESOLUTION
Knowledge of the donor's wishes
Attributes of the donor
Personal realisation of death
Confirmation of death
Information about retrieval

Saying goodbye
'What do I do now?'

RESOLUTION
Options and advice
about 'saying goodbye'
Post retrieval telephone call

CONFLICT

Leaving a person who does
not appear to be dead
Aesthetic presentation of the body

Dealing with grief
and donation

CONFLICT

Termination of the affectional
bonds for parts of the relative
that live on
Donation decisions
Lack of bereavement support

RESOLUTION
Focusing on the achievement
of the donor
Information about the
recipients
Feeling of making a
contribution
Knowing some good has
come out of the death
The donation is recognised,
valued and not forgotten
Specialist bereavement
support

BST= Brainstem tests

compounded by a lack of experience and knowledge about the process of organ donation:

Oh, the whole thing was something quite new. (12)

The above participant's reaction cannot be considered unusual, as deaths in situations where organ donation is a possibility remain rare events. For instance, an audit of all deaths in 341 UK intensive care units from 1 April 2003–31 March 2005 showed that of 46,801 dead patients, 2740 were potential heartbeating organ donors; 1244 of whom became donors (Barber *et al.* 2006). The inexperience of families living through these phenomena must also be weighed against the 600,000 deaths per annum in the UK (Hicks and Allen 1999). These figures make it clear that it is unlikely that a family will ever have experienced the particular circumstances of organ donation. Health care professionals can therefore expect that families more often than not have had no role models for their decision-making and possess no discrete knowledge or experience of the process of organ donation. Yet it is within this environment that they are asked to make complex decisions about donation that may have implications for their own emotional well-being and ability to cope with their bereavement.

However, studies indicate that importance is attributed to relatives' need to consider organ or tissue donation (Manninen and Evans 1985; Sque 1996; Sque and Wells 2004; Sque *et al.* 2005). Relatives who were asked felt that they probably would not have thought of organ donation and were glad they were approached. They felt it would have been distressing not to be able to fulfil the pre-mortem wish of the donor. Alternatively Featherstone (1994), Pelletier (1993a) and Finlay and Dallimore (1991), report the distress caused when families were not given this option. Relatives felt that their loved one's organs had been wasted and that they were denied the opportunity to have some good come from their loss.

Callahan (1987) points out that the expressed wishes of the dead generally merit respect in their own right. This may help to explain the gratitude that was felt by relatives who were asked about donation and were able to facilitate the wish of the donor; a finding supported by Pelletier (1993a). It was also shown by Douglass and Daly (1995), Pelletier (1993b) and Tymstra *et al.* (1992), that knowing that they had made a worthwhile contribution comforted relatives. Therefore, because of the importance attached to the wishes of the dead, and the action that relatives are able to take on their behalf, it seems imperative that next of kin[2] should be given the option to facilitate donation.

These findings suggest that in situations of a donor's clinical suitability efforts need to be made to discuss organ donation with relatives. Health care professionals need to be aware, and feel confident that relatives are most likely to be grateful that the option of donation was discussed with them (Sque 1996; Sque *et al.* 2003).

Realizing

Becoming aware things are going wrong – realization of death

The time between the social acceptance of death and the objective confirmation of death was shown to be especially difficult for participants, as they privately questioned their convictions of death occurring and experienced difficulties in coping with the enquiries of friends and family. For instance, they now felt uncomfortable talking to and interacting with what they perceived to be a ventilated corpse. One participant had been told that her son would not recover but that she had to wait for confirmation of death. During this time she found it difficult to keep up the charade that he was still alive, when dealing with enquiries of relatives and friends. She reported:

> That was the worse bit, the hanging around, because they had to get rid of the drugs or something, and you know in the papers [report in the local newspaper] it's, 'stable', 'critical', we know he is dead, and people coming up, 'I hope he gets better', you know, and you can't say anything as such, but you know he has gone, and it was Tuesday 1 o'clock they certified him as dead. I think that was the worse bit, that sort of 24 hours from the time he had gone, to the time they could officially announce, yes, he's dead. (03)

These events led some participants to desire an early end to the perceived suffering of their relative with the confirmation of death:

> I couldn't see A lying in the bed in that condition being artificially kept alive, although I no longer, I no longer believed he was alive, I just believed that his body was functioning and so, I wanted to see him released from that. (16)

Therefore healthcare professionals need to be aware of families' distress when interacting with ventilated, potential donors, thus the need not to delay the confirmation of death.

Deciding

Confirmation of brainstem death

Within the context of bereavement, donor relatives faced with a tragic and sudden death are at high risk of aberrant bereavement outcomes (Yates *et al.* 1990; Wright 1996; Stroebe and Schut 2002). The unexpected nature of the death may make its acceptance difficult for families to reconcile. Next of kin are necessarily approached about organ donation when their grief may be all encompassing and thinking and concentration a problem. However, if donation is to take place families need to make a number of decisions on behalf of their deceased relative. These decisions may be problematic, as they concern an operation on another's body; yet, the time to debate the issues is limited. Relatives are asked to accept a non-traditional death, brainstem death, as death. The implications of brainstem death transcend the usual experience of the lay individual. The potential donor maintained on a ventilator may not look dead, and often has no external manifestations of injury. They tend to be unscathed, resting, warm, florid and their chest moves as if they are breathing; they may even move occasionally if a spinal reflex is activated. Their time of death becomes an arbitrary decision made by the attending physicians. Not only are relatives asked to accept this situation as death, but also they are asked to agree to the removal of the very vital organs that normally would maintain life. Appropriate explanations of how clinical neurological tests confirm death appeared to be important to relatives, as well as the opportunity to attend brainstem testing.

It was shown that the lack of knowledge and explanation about these events can cause families considerable distress, while attending brainstem testing and receiving information in caring, timely and complementary ways may be helpful to some relatives (Sque *et al.* 2005; Long *et al.* 2006).

Three families experienced further difficulties when told conflicting times of death. Participants found a number of ways to deal with this complex issue; some decided not to see the ventilated relative once death was confirmed. Others had confidence in the outcome of brainstem tests, which appeared to be coupled with their own sense of death already occurring. Others were reassured by visiting with the body after the donation operation. A participant gave a description of her experience when she saw her son in the chapel of rest:

> A reassuring experience, made it final, as it was difficult to accept death, when in hospital he just looked as if he was sleeping. (03)

Families of ventilated, major organ donors need to be given unambiguous information about the time of death. The time of death for organ donors is when death is conclusively established and no other time (Department of Health Working Party 1998).[3]

Donation decisions

Conflict continued for participants throughout the process of decision-making about donation; deciding if donation should take place, and which organs or tissues should be donated. Decisions about donation were mainly consensus family decisions. Four resolutions appeared important to participants in their deliberations (see Table 4.2).

Table 4.2 Influences on donation decisions

Wishes of the deceased known	Wishes of the deceased unknown
Discussion with relatives	
Carried a donor card/wish known	Attributes of the deceased
Personal realization of death	
Confirmation of brainstem death	
To help others	
Not to just switch the ventilator off	
To fulfil the needs of the family members	
To give meaning to the donor's life	

Reprinted from *Social Science & Medicine*, 49(3): Sque, M. and Payne, S., Dissonant loss: the experiences of donor relatives, 1359–70 (1996) with permission from Elsevier.

These were the knowledge of the donor's wishes, the attributes of the donor, clinical confirmation of death and a personal realization of death: A wife said:

> I was stroking his arm and he was lovely and warm and then I touched his hand, and that always sticks in my mind how cold his hands suddenly went. I knew there was something wrong, I knew he wasn't, I knew he wasn't coming home, put it that way. (05)

Personal motivations also played a part in participants' willingness to facilitate donation:

> It's selfish really, because I wanted him to go on. I wanted a bit of him to go on living, you see. (15)

Special sentiment was attributed to the heart and eyes (Helman 1991; Wells and Sque 2002), which were respectively the least donated organ and tissue. A wife said:

> He always drew hearts with arrows through them and that, and I thought I can't, it didn't seem right for me to let somebody else have his heart ... I couldn't the heart. (15)

It was very important to participants that retrieval was carried out with dignity and propriety and their relative did not suffer. Poor knowledge of the procedure for the donation operation also raised concern:

> We don't know what they done or how they did it or where they did it, or, there was just no one, just come and say anything about it all. Did they up to this day? We still haven't got a clue, you know. (11)

Relatives have to depend on information given to them by medical and nursing staff. It is therefore worth considering the pressure that may be implicitly exerted on relatives, in terms of the type of information and its timeliness to fit in with the overall prevailing atmosphere within the intensive care unit at the time. The atmosphere could depend on the workload and the degree to which staff share in the philosophy of providing care for patients who are not likely to recover. Lipshitz (1993) highlighted the importance imposed by environments in which decisions are made, both in terms of understanding the decision and the strategies followed, which are influenced by the perceptions of the decision-maker. Moritsugu (1998) has also stressed the importance of the 'peri-donation' environment and need for the family to feel nurtured and supported in their grief.

Parting

Saying goodbye

An opportunity to say, 'goodbye', and share in the final moments of a loved one's life has been documented by several authors to be important to many. Deep resentment can be felt among families when it was perceived that such an opportunity had been denied (Seale and Kelly 1997). Parting and making the decision to leave the ventilated relative (who did not appear to be dead) produced a poignant conflict for participants. Although they had recognized the relative's death, their appearance was incongruent with participants' expectations of the appearance of a dead body. Resolutions to this conflict concerned the traditional accepted nature of death, such as knowledge of the cessation of the heartbeat, or viewing the still, pale, dead body post the donation operation. Sometimes nurses offered to inform participants when the donation operation was complete. Some participants found the time waiting for this telephone call, and the declaration of cessation of the heartbeat, difficult. On the one hand, it marked a kind of finality but it was an end to any hope of existence for the relative. A wife explains:

> We got the phone call 4.30 Christmas Eve to say they had switched off the ventilator. That was terrible waiting for the phone call. We dreaded the phone to ring, I mean, we knew that he had gone then. (15)

Some participants were offered the facility of visiting their relative in the chapel of rest and accepted the opportunity to do so. Participants were given an appointment for the day following the donation operation and told to report to the main reception in the hospital where they were directed to the chapel of rest. They were then left to visit, unsupported. They were often distressed by what they saw and many regretted this encounter. Being relatively young, some participants had never seen a dead body. A mother and father were 'shocked' when they saw their daughter, as they were previously unaware that her eyes had been removed. Participants, also, had many unanswered questions at this time, which was a continuing source of worry and speculation. A lack of preparation led to distressing fantasies as this participant reported about her visit to a chapel of rest:

> I just kept thinking if they lifted up that blanket what would they find? (11)

Participants felt that there was much room for improvement of this service. They felt that some preparation for what they were to see in the chapel of rest could have been helpful, as well as being accompanied by a health care professional they knew. In no case did hospitals offer participants a full range of options for seeing the relative post donation, such as back in the intensive care unit, which might have been appropriate for some. This did cause regrets among participants, as they felt viewing the newly-dead would have been preferable rather than (sometimes) days later at a funeral home:

> Perhaps if after you have donated these organs, then perhaps if the hospital rang you and said, right would you like to come back now and see them, perhaps that would be better, because it is not so long is it? Five days is a long time really. (05)

Retrospectively, participants wished that they had more guidance from hospital staff about options and the possible effects of choosing how and when they said goodbye. When this advice was given, participants were very grateful. A young mother reported:

> She [nurse] said, 'Many people that don't hold their babies regrets it later on'. 'Why don't you hold him?' I said, 'Oh, I don't know', and she reassured me that you know, it was the best thing to do. So I did and I can't thank her enough, I am so glad that I held him for that last time, held him twice actually, in that same night, and I am so glad that I did, I think she is right, I would have regretted it not holding him for that last time, I felt so chuffed, I felt so proud, my baby. I didn't see him in the chapel of rest or anything like that, because I had actually held him, you know, in my arms and everything and that was my last experience of him. (08)

There is a need for guidance and choice to be provided by health care professionals about the options and the possible effects of choosing how and when relatives 'say goodbye' to organ donors. I suggest that it would be helpful for relatives to have the support of a health care professional known to them during the visit to the chapel of rest. This person could discuss with relatives what to expect in terms of the setting and the presentation of the donor. Coupe (1991) stated that relatives said they were not given enough advice about how the body would look (particularly, with major organ donors, who will be very pale, due to the exsanguination of virtually their entire blood volume). It would give the health care professional a chance to view the body first, and make sure it was in an acceptable condition to be visited; for instance, if eyes had been removed, that the face looks as natural as possible, this being important to relatives. Both Bradbury (1999) and Verble and Worth (2000) have remarked that cultural expectations have an impact on the aesthetic presentation of the dead, which could be assumed to be particularly important with young donors. Such interaction could also be helpful to health care professionals, as they would be able to complete the cycle of care, shown to be desirable for job satisfaction (Borozny 1990; Watson 1991). The possible benefits of post donation visiting need to be considered as part of complete bereavement care (see Chapter 2) but relatives need preparation and support for visits with organ donors.

'What do I do now?'

A father asked intensive care staff as he was about to leave the unit: 'What do I do now?'. The question indicates the bewildering stage of leaving hospital and dealing with immediate concerns of the death and its outcome. Hospitals generally did not provide advice about grief, give bereavement support contacts or carry out follow-up. Only in two cases did consultants and transplant coordinators suggest participants should get in touch if they had unanswered questions. A 'debrief' opportunity with hospital staff or a transplant co-ordinator to discuss any remaining concerns such as issues about brainstem testing, the diagnosis of the critical illness or the trajectory of the illness was shown to be desired by families, and has been adopted in some institutions (Sque *et al.* 2006).

Coping

Dealing with grief and donation

Conflicts continued for participants throughout their bereavement process. These conflicts concerned the incompatible notions of the continuance of the life of the donated organs with the reality of the donor's death. Resolutions to these grief conflicts were provided when information was available to participants about the outcome and continued contribution of the donation. A lack of skilled bereavement support and pertinent information appeared to compound some participants' distress. Due to the mainly sudden, untimely and non-traditional nature of donors' death, relatives are at high risk of aberrant bereavement. Therefore, a need exists for bereavement follow-up and support for donor families. It may be useful for transplant coordinating services and hospitals to consider how these bereavement needs may be met, moving with the family from the bedside into the community setting.

The most important thing about grief and donation is that donation does not appear to make grief any less (Cleiren and Van Zoelen 2002), but for some participants it changed the emphasis of death to focus on the achievement of the donor (Sque and Payne 1996).

Participants reported that the greatest respite from grief was the ability to talk to others, when they needed to, about their bereavement. Participants tended to seek out their own social supports but grief was largely managed within the family. A few participants who did not have family support sought the help of bereavement organizations, who seemed ill-prepared to be of assistance in this particular circumstance. Families who used bereavement services did not feel that the experiences had been particularly helpful. In one case, the counsellor expressed her objection to organ donation!

Participants received a letter within two weeks of the donation from the transplant coordinating services, which gave some information about organ distribution. They found this initial information helpful but desired more about recipients:

> In some ways it would be nice to know more specifically what hap-pened to P's organs. They gave a general scenario, but the problem in this case, it was that this person was doing OK but if they gave a little

LIVERPOOL JOHN MOORES UNIVERSITY
LEARNING SERVICES

description, what people are like [participant suggests] a P.E. teacher who had a heart problem is back teaching, in that sense I guess it would be nice if one had more information. (04)

There is a need for recognition of relatives' desire for particular information about recipients, and the benefits they receive from donated organs (Sque 2000; Holtkamp 2002). Although the letter from the transplant coordinating service was helpful, and some participants did receive a letter from the organ recipients, there was, generally, a desire for continued information on the progress of recipients; and participants were disappointed when further follow-up was not available (Sque 2000). This appeared to be important in resolving the conflict of having a part of their relative still living on:

> Would like to be kept informed how recipients are doing ... comfort to us to know that part of J is still doing some good to different people. (11)

The desire for information did not necessarily abate as time went by. A mother interviewed at 36 months still felt:

> As time goes by I would like to know more. (12)

In some cases, participants realized that they may not wish to know if the transplant had failed. Others thought this was unimportant as, at least, help had been offered. Participants were comforted by the knowledge that they helped to facilitate a worthwhile contribution:

> We were chatting about transplants funnily enough, because it wasn't long after N died and everything, a matter of weeks. Something came on the telly about donors and that relief that I felt, you know, that we'd actually done something. (08)

At the time of the interview, although some participants had experienced difficulties with aspects of their bereavement, all remained supportive of their donation decision:

> No concern at all, chuffed as hell. (02)

Although the efficacy of bereavement interventions has recently been questioned (Schut *et al.* 2002) there is evidence to suggest that social support and professional help remain important to individuals, like some donor relatives, who may be at risk of poor bereavement outcomes (Walter 1996; Payne *et al.* 1999; Riches and Dawson 2000; Holtkamp 2002). The Conference of Medical Royal Colleges and their Faculties in the UK as long ago as 1987 recommended that health authorities should recognize that organ donor families may have certain bereavement needs. Clearly, some participants in this study needed support; but of a particular kind. Unfortunately, many failed to receive the help they needed and sometimes interactions with bereavement counsellors were deleterious. The study showed that general bereavement counsellors seemed ill-prepared to help participants. There appears to be a need for bereavement services to develop services to effectively support donor families.

It was a desire of participants that their relatives' contribution was recognized, valued and not forgotten. Simple forms of this recognition could be 'books of remembrance' kept in hospitals. A more elaborate form of memorial could be a dedicated garden or an 'eternal flame'. What is important is that these memorials could, respectively, be given a place of prominence in hospitals, or in an important national park. This not only recognizes the humanitarian contribution of the donation but could help to promote public education about organ and tissue donation (Sque 1995). While there is no evidence of the effect of bereavement anniversary cards for donor families, Hutchison (1995) found anniversary cards to be comforting and supportive to survivors of patients who died in a hospice.

Nurses' and doctors' own awareness and education about the donation of organs and tissues needs to be guided by the above ideals; also, national and local health care policies. Of particular importance appears to be the experience of caring for donors and their significant others as Maloney and Altmaier (2003) highlight the continuing difficulties health care professionals have with managing the affective responses of the bereaved family. Issues regarding death, dying and the management of the dead body in modern western society may usefully underpin organ donation education. The historical impact of traditional values regarding death is fundamental to these issues. Time needs to be allocated for health care professionals to reflect upon their own feelings about donation and transplantation. Where it is appropriate, health care staff need to be educated to recognize donors and approach families about donation. Issues of particular importance appear to be the timing and nature of the donation discussion (Sque *et al.* 2003, 2006; Rodrique *et al.* 2006). This should always be carried out in a manner to facilitate a decision by the next of kin that will not be regretted (see Chapter 5).

Hospitals should have policies to identify potential donors and to inform families of their option to donate. Effective policies are needed to support staff so that donation discussions are not left to individual preferences. This would mean that hospitals need to consider systems for documenting that donation was discussed with the next of kin; have a duty to educate staff about donation; and should monitor the impact of donation discussions on the overall availability of organs and tissues for transplantation.

Critique of the theory

The research approach allowed, even with a small sample, a substantive theoretical perspective to be derived, which helps to explain donor families' experiences and relationships between concepts, to provide a framework for making predictions. While caution must be exerted in the findings from a small sample and each participant's experience remains unique to them, it is likely that many aspects of their experience will be common to others.

Primarily, one of the exemplar contributions and strengths of this theory is that it was developed from data that provided the families' perceptions of the donation experience, narrated by them and reflecting their worldview. Therefore, it is expected to have relevance to the study of other individuals in similar circumstances. A weakness in the theoretical construction is that participants were interviewed only once as donor relatives' needs and perceptions of their experiences could change over time. However, a longitudinal study (Sque *et al.* 2003) has verified and extended the theoretical premises of this study. As has work with families who chose not to donate organs of their deceased relatives (Sque *et al.* 2006).

I am a nurse committed to the donation process. This does raise the question about the nature of the information collected and its interpretation. My professional background undoubtedly had an impact on the interaction with participants and the development and pursuance of the research agenda, and is a source of bias. However, my professional knowledge and intimate acquaintance with hospital protocol and procedures involving donors gave me a particular ability to critically analyse the interview data in terms of professional responsibilities and the lived experience of organ donation.

A criticism of the research outcome could be that the theory and conceptual model produced are monolithic and one-dimensional and do not take account of diversity; the data being embedded in the traditional values and prevailing contemporary death culture of western society. However, the outcomes of research will tend to be evaluated in terms of its persuasiveness and the power to inspire an audience (Pidgeon and Henwood 1997). In this regard, the theory suggests a number of potentially useful interpretations.

Making the donation experience explicit may contribute to an understanding of the psychosocial issues involved in organ donation. The theory suggests areas where help may be focused. An increased understanding of the needs of participants could provide indicators for the appropriate care of other populations of donor relatives and a theoretical foundation for the education of health care professionals. The theory provides a plausible groundwork for continued research with populations we clearly know little about, such as those relatives who refuse donation. The investigation has provided supportive evidence for other studies concerning donor relatives

(Simmonds *et al.* 1987; Buckley 1989; Savaria *et al.* 1990; Tymstra *et al.* 1992; La Spina *et al.* 1993; Pelletier 1993a, 1993b; Cleiren and Van Zoelen 2002; Sque *et al.* 2003, 2005; Ormrod *et al.* 2005; Rodrique *et al.* 2006).

Glaser and Strauss (1967) and Glaser (2005) view theory very much as process. Therefore, the theory needs to be subjected to further refinement and elaboration. The fittingness and robustness of this theoretical perspective lends itself to replication and exploration in other sites, with different samples and patient populations. The theory provides the opportunity to generate new ideas, suggest the inferences and hypotheses that can be formulated from them and suggest the direction and growth of research. Although the derived categories were perceived important for this group of donor relatives, the theory identified is open to support or refutation by other investigators. Similar research questions need to be asked and consideration given to the researcher's perspective, if comparable findings are desirable. The theory could usefully be applied to other situations of loss that involve conflicts and complex decision-making, such as in mutilating, elective surgery, or decision-making about disconnecting patients from life-support, or terminating curative medical treatment.

I believe that one of the major ontological contributions of the theory of dissonant loss is that it has explicated, for the first time, a comprehensive account of families' experiences of organ donation, and that this has been achieved within the particular social context of the UK. Not only has an explanation of these events been provided but the core category of conflict and resolution was identified, which makes the other categories within the theory even more valid because of their integral cohesiveness and consistency.

Conclusion

This chapter has attempted to address the paucity of information and theoretical support needed to further an understanding of the donation process, to provide effective, appropriate methods, to support donor relatives in their bereavement and health care professionals in their difficult work. A study that suggested that relatives' experience of organ donation could be explained through a theory of dissonant loss has been described. Conflict existed for relatives in two particular forms during the donation process. On the one hand conflict existed as a series of events over which relatives had no control, such as the ambiguity of brainstem death. Other conflicts emerged through decisions that needed to be made about donation. These decisions tended to take place in a highly charged emotional environment. The theory suggests areas where help may be focused and may usefully be applied to other situations of loss that involve conflicts and complex decision-making. Clearly, there is still a lot we do not yet understand or know about the donation process and its psychosocial effects. Dissonant loss theory may provide a framework for further investigation.

Acknowledgements

The research upon which this chapter is based was supported by a British Department of Health Nursing Research Studentship.

Notes

1 'The last time we were together'; 'finding out something is wrong'; 'waiting for a diagnosis'; and 'hopes and expectations' contained, respectively, information about participants' early experiences of the critical illness or injury. For further information about these categories readers are advised to see Sque, M. (2001) Being a carer in acute crisis: the situation for relatives of organ donors, in S. Payne and C. Ellis-Hill (eds) *Chronic and Terminal Illness: New Perspectives on Caring and Carers*. Oxford: Oxford University Press.

2 In the UK Human Tissue Act (2004) states in Part 1, Section 2 that in the case of a child 'appropriate consent means the consent of a person who has parental responsibility for him [the child]'. Section 3 states that in the case of an adult 'appropriate consent' rests with 'a nominated person' or 'person who stood in a qualifying relationship to him immediately before he died'. This person may not be the next of kin. There are a number of criteria given defining a nominated person and a qualifying relationship.

3 The Code of Practice for Diagnosis and Certification of Death is presently under review by a Working Party of the Royal College of Anaesthetists in the UK on behalf of the Academy of Medical Royal Colleges and the English Department of Health.

References

Bradbury, M. (1999) *Representations of Death: A Social Psychological Perspective*. London: Routledge.

Buckley, P. (1989) Donor family surveys provide useful information for organ procurement, *Transplantation Proceedings*, 21(1): 1411–12.

Callahan, J.C. (1987) Harming the dead, *Ethics*, 97: 341–52.

Cleiren, M.P.H.D. and Van Zoelen, A.J. (2002) Post mortem organ donation and grief: a study of consent, refusal and well-being in bereavement, *Death Studies*, 26: 837–49.

Conference of Medical Royal Colleges and their Faculties in the United Kingdom. (1987) *Report of the Working Party on the Supply of Donor Organs for Transplantation*. London: HMSO.

Coupe, D. (1991) *A study of relatives' nurses' and doctors' attitudes of the support and information given to the families of potential organ donors*. M.Phil. thesis, University of Wales College of Medicine, Cardiff, UK.

Department of Health Working Party (1998) *A Code of Practice for the Diagnosis of Brain Stem Death*. London: HMSO.

Douglass, G.E. and Daly, M. (1995) Donor families' experience of organ donation, *Anaesthesia and Intensive Care*, 23(1): 96–8.

Featherstone, K. (1994) Nurses' knowledge and attitudes toward organ and tissue donation in a community hospital, *Journal of Trauma Nursing*, 1(2): 57–63.

Finlay, I. and Dallimore, D. (1991) Your child is dead, *British Medical Journal*, 302: 1524–5.

Glaser, B. (2005) *The Grounded Theory Perspective III: Theoretical Coding*. Mill Valley: Sociology Press.

Glaser, B. and Strauss, A. (1967) *Discovery of Grounded Theory*. Chicago: Aldine.

Helman, C. (1991) *Body Myths*. London: Chatto & Windus.

Hicks, J. and Allen, G. (1999) *A Century of Change: Trends in UK Statistics since 1900*, Research paper 99/111. London: House of Commons Library.

Holtkamp, S. (2002) *Wrapped in Mourning: The Gift of Life and Organ Donor Family Trauma*. New York: Brunner-Routledge.

Hutchinson, S.M. (1995) Evaluation of bereavement anniversary cards, *Journal of Palliative Care*, 11(3): 32–4.

La Spina, F., Sedda, L., Pizzi, C., Verlato, R., Boselli, L., Candiani, A., Chiaranda, M., Frova, G., Gorgerino, F., Gravame, V., Mapelli, A., Martini, C., Pappalettera, M., Seveso, M. and Sironi, P.G. (1993) Donor families' attitude toward organ donation, *Transplantation Proceedings*, 25(1): 1699–701.

Lipshitz, R. (1993) Converging themes in the study of decision making in realistic settings, in G.A. Klein, J. Orasanu, R. Calderwood and C.E. Zsambok (eds) *Decision-making in Action: Models and Methods*. Norwood, NJ: Ablex.

Long, T., Sque, M. and Payne, S. (2006) Information sharing: its impact on donor and non-donor families' experiences in hospital, *Progress in Transplantation*, 16(2): 144–9.

Maloney, R. and Altmaier, E.M. (2003) Caring for bereaved families: self-efficacy in the donation request process, *Journal of Clinical Psychology in Medical Settings*, 10: 251–8.

Manninen, D.L. and Evans, R.W. (1985) Public attitudes and behaviour regarding organ donation, *Journal of the American Medical Association*, 253(21): 3111–15.

Moritsugu, K. (1998) Pay attention to the peri-donation environment. Coalition on Donation Progress notes Archive, www.transweb.org/partnership/prog_notes/spring98/pn_spring98.htlm#dr (accessed June 2005).

Ormrod, J.A., Ryder, T., Chadwick, R.J. and Bonner. S.M. (2005) Experiences of families when a relative is diagnosed brain stem dead: understanding of death, observation of brain stem death testing and attitudes to organ donation, *Anaesthesia*, 60: 1002–8.

Payne, S., Horn, S. and Relf, M. (1999) *Loss and Bereavement*. Buckingham: Open University Press.

Pelletier, M. (1993a) The needs of family members of organ and tissue donors, *Heart & Lung*, 22(2): 151–7.

Pelletier, M. (1993b) Emotions experienced and coping strategies used by family members of organ donors, *Canadian Journal of Nursing Research*, 25(2): 63–73.

Pigeon, N. and Henwood, K. (1997) Using grounded theory in psychological research, in N. Hayes (ed.) *Qualitative Analysis in Psychology*. Hove: Psychology Press.

Riches, G. and Dawson, P. (2000) *An Intimate Loneliness: Supporting Bereaved Parents and Siblings*. Buckingham: Open University Press.

Rodrique, J.R., Cornell, D.L. and Howard, R.J. (2006) Organ donation decision: comparision of donor and non-donor families, *American Journal of Transplantation*, 6: 190–8.

Savaria, D.T., Rovelli, M.A. and Schweizer, R.T. (1990) Donor family surveys provide useful information for organ procurement, *Transplantation Proceedings*, 22(2): 316–17.

Schut, H., Stroebe, M.S., Van den Bout, J. and Terheggen, M. (2002) The efficacy of bereavement interventions: determining the benefits, in M.S. Stroebe, R.O. Hansson, W. Stroebe and H. Schut (eds) *Handbook of Bereavement Research: Consequences, Coping, and Care*. Washington, DC: American Psychological Association.

Seale, C. and Kelly, M. (1997) A comparison of hospice and hospital care for people who die: views of surviving spouses, *Palliative Medicine*, 11: 101–6.

Simmons, R.G., Marine, S.K. and Simmons, R.L. (eds) (1987) *Gift of Life: The Effect of Organ Transplantation on Individual, Family, and Societal Dynamics*. New Brunswick, NJ: Transaction Books.

Sque, M. (1995) Feature: transplant services, organ donation Miami style, *Nursing Standard*, 42: 8–20.

Sque, M. (1996) *The experiences of donor relatives, and nurses' attitudes, knowledge and behaviour regarding cadaveric donotransplantation*. Ph.D. thesis, University of Southampton, Southampton: UK.

Sque, M. (2000) *'A Story to Tell': Post Bereavement Correspondence Between Organ Donor Families, Recipients, Their OPOs and the National Donor Family Council – An American Investigation*. A report of a study funded by The General Nursing Council for England & Wales Trust. University of Surrey, Guildford: UK.

Sque, M. and Payne, S. (1996) Dissonant loss: the experiences of donor relatives, *Social Science & Medicine*, 43(9): 1359–70.

Sque, M. and Wells, J. (2004) Organ donation: helping patients and families make choices, in S. Payne, J. Seymour and I. Ingleton (eds) *Palliative Care Nursing: Principles and Evidence for Practice*. Maidenhead: Open University Press.

Sque, M., Long, T. and Payne, S. (2003) *Organ and Tissue Donation: Exploring the Needs of Families*. Final report of a three-year study commissioned by the British Organ Donor Society, funded by the Community Fund. University of Southampton, Southampton: UK.

Sque, M., Long, T. and Payne, S. (2005) Organ donation: key factors influencing families' decision-making, *Transplantation Proceedings*, 37: 543–6.

Sque, M., Long, T., Payne, S. and Allardyce, D. (2006) *Exploring the End of Life Decision-making and Hospital Experiences of Families Who Did Not Donate Organs or Tissues for Transplant Operations*. Final report for UK Transplant. University of Southampton, Southampton: UK.

Stroebe, W. and Schut, H. (2002) Risk factors in bereavement outcome: a methodological and empirical review, in M.S. Stroebe, R.O. Hansson, W. Stroebe and H. Schut (eds) *Handbook of Bereavement Research: Consequences, Coping, and Care*. Washington, DC: American Psychological Association.

Tymstra, Tj., Heyink, J.W., Pruim, J. and Slooff, M.J.H. (1992) Experience of bereaved relatives who granted or refused permission for organ donation, *Family Practice*, 9(2): 141–4.

Verble, M. and Worth, J. (2000) Fears and concerns expressed by families in the donation discussion, *Progress in Transplantation*, 10: 48–55.

Walter, T. (1996) A new model of grief, *Mortality*, 1(1): 7–25.

Watson, K. (1991) Developing positive attitudes to procurement surgery, *ACORN Journal*, 4(6): 31–6.

Wells, J. and Sque, M. (2002) 'Living choice': the commitment to tissue donation in palliative care, *International Journal of Palliative Nursing*, 8(1): 22–7.

Wright, B. (1996) *Sudden Death: A Research Base for Practice*, 2nd edn. New York: Churchill Livingstone.

Yates, D.W., Ellison, G. and McGuiness, S. (1990) Care of the suddenly bereaved, *British Medical Journal*, 301: 29–31.

5 Supporting families' decision-making about organ donation

Tracy Long

Introduction

This chapter explores the experiences of family members during their hospital stay, from admission, through the confirmation of death using brainstem testing to the request for organ donation. It considers the approach and discussion about organ donation with the aim of identifying factors that may support family members as they make decisions regarding donation. The chapter will draw upon a three-year longitudinal study carried out by Sque *et al.* (2003) as well as research selected from the last 15 years.

End of life decisions remain with the living long after the death of a family member and have been implicated in abnormal and complicated grief (Saunders 1993; Wright 1996). As families have a time-limited opportunity to consider organ donation, it is imperative that the approach and discussion about donation by health professionals facilitates a decision that will not be regretted later (Burroughs *et al.* 1998). In their study examining the psychological consequences of consenting or refusing organ and tissue donation, Burroughs *et al.* (1998: 161) reported that 21 per cent of their sample of 159 donating and 66 non-donating family members 'indicated that they would not make the same decision again', that in fact they were dissatisfied with their decision. How do we ensure that people are satisfied with their decision regarding organ donation and that they leave the hospital comfortable with the decision they made in the most difficult of situations, the sudden unexpected death of a relative, and not just a sudden death but a death that is diagnosed using neurological criteria?

Death diagnosed by brainstem testing

Neurological death, whether it be whole-brain death (USA) or brainstem death (UK)[1] is a prerequisite for cadaveric organ donation (unless donation of livers and kidneys follows circulatory arrest) and is therefore a fundamental factor in the process of organ and tissue donation for transplantation. Testing carried out to confirm cessation of all brainstem functions (UK) or whole-brain function (USA) is required to certify death, if the death is based on neurological criteria (Powner and Darby 1999). As death based on neurological criteria is a relatively recent development that has resulted in two further criteria, one based on a whole-brain function and the other on brainstem function, a brief history of its development will follow.

Historical background to the development of the concept 'brain death'

Historically relevant to the development of the concept of brain death were reports coming out of France in the late 1950s. Neurosurgeons in Lyon reported the 'death of the nervous system' (Wertheimer *et al.* 1959), a condition characterized by persistent apnoea, coma, absent brainstem and tendon reflexes and an electrically silent brain (Pallis 1994). Patients diagnosed with this condition had a pulse as long as respiratory ventilation was maintained, but there was no spontaneous respiration if mechanical ventilation was stopped. Later the same year a more detailed account of the same condition was published by Mollaret and Goulon (1959). They described 'a state beyond coma' and called this state *coma dépassé*. *Coma dépassé* defined a syndrome, whereby a patient's heart and lung functions could be maintained, but in which there was loss of all reflexes and all brain activity, and where consciousness never returned. Therefore a patient who had lost all brain activity could be kept functioning by artificial ventilation, intravenous feeding and other intensive care interventions (Haupt and Rudolf 1999).

   This situation raised a number of issues that were influential in the development of neurological criteria for diagnosing death:

- When could doctors discontinue 'futile' treatment, such as the maintenance of severely brain damaged patients on artificial ventilators, patients who, in the view of the medical physician, would not recover?
- When was the moment of death, as this influenced the status of the deceased from a legal standpoint? Isolating a moment of death changes a person's legal status in relation to certain rights, claims and entitlements. When can the will be enacted, and in the USA, when can medical insurance companies stop paying for the care of the ventilated patient?
- Being able to indicate the moment of death was a crucial issue for those medical practitioners who felt that patients sustained on ventilators were a valuable source of viable organs for transplantation. Surgeons working in renal transplantation had already

commented on the benefits of kidneys from cadavers (Tilney 2003), but without a fixed time point of death doctors ran the risk of being charged with murder as removing the heart or kidneys from a seriously ill patient would certainly result in their death.

In response to these issues, a committee of experts was convened at the Harvard Medical School in 1968. The Harvard Committee presented a report that outlined guidelines for the diagnosis of a state called 'irreversible coma'. Their report recommended that irreversible coma should be accepted as equivalent to death (Ad Hoc Committee of the Harvard Medical School 1968). The Harvard report did not mention organ donation or transplantation; in fact the Harvard Committee had tried to disassociate the issue of a new definition of death and organ transplantation, but the link was made at the 22nd World Medical Assembly in August of 1968 where the issue of organ transplantation was a particular topic of debate. The Harvard guidelines were corroborated by this conference and resulted in the Sydney Declaration, which affirmed the medical view that death was a process, and that brain death could be clinically established.

Once brain death could be clinically established in ventilator dependent patients, the whole issue of removing organs for transplantation (organs that had not suffered the deleterious effects of circulatory cessation) gained impetus. In the USA there were concerns within the medical professions regarding potential civil and criminal outcomes of organ donation procedures and therefore a review of the legal status of the Harvard criteria of brain death was carried out by the medical consultants of the President's Commission for the Study of Ethical Problems in Medicine Biochemical and Behavioral Research (Capron 1999). This resulted in a report entitled *Defining Death* (President's Commission 1981), which sought to reach a consensus definition that would provide the accepted medical standards by which all patients would be measured. The updated guidelines provided by the Commission, supported both a cardiopulmonary standard *and* a neurological standard for diagnosing death and are detailed in the Uniform Determination of Death Act 1981 (UDDA), which states that 'an individual who has sustained either 1) irreversible cessation of circulatory and respiratory functions or 2) irreversible cessation of all functions of the entire brain, including the brainstem, is dead' and that 'a determination of death must be made in accordance with accepted medical standard' (President's Commission 1981: 119).

The UDDA had been adopted by all US states and brain death is recognized as legal death in all states. While this criterion has been adopted by other countries around the world, it is not the criteria applied in the UK.

In 1976, the Conference of Medical Royal Colleges and their Faculties in the UK (Working Group) published a memorandum called the 'Diagnosis of brain death' which laid out a tripartite prognostic criteria for the purpose of justifying the action of removing 'hopeless' cases from mechanical support (Evans and Potts 2000).

The conference memorandum stated that brain death 'is accepted as being sufficient to distinguish between those patients who retain the functional capacity to have a chance of even partial recovery from those in whom no such possibility exists' (Working Group 1976: 1187). The 1976 memorandum did not state that brain death was death and therefore in 1979 the 1976 recommendations were updated in a memorandum of the Working Group called 'Diagnosis of death' and as the title suggests the aim was to equate the death of the brain with the death of the individual. Therefore, what had been, initially, prognostic criteria became diagnostic criteria (Evans and Potts 2000).

As with the Harvard guidelines, neither the 1976 nor the 1979 memorandums specifically referred to organ transplantation, but when these memoranda were incorporated into a document, published by the Department of Health of Great Britain and Northern Ireland in 1983 called '*Cadaveric Organs for Transplantation: A Code of Practice Including the Diagnosis of Brain Death*', the connection between brain death and organ donation was made. This connection was then made explicit and standardized by the publication in 1998, again by the Department of Health of *A Code of Practice for the Diagnosis of Brain Stem Death: Including Guidelines for the Identification and Management of Potential Organ and Tissue Donors.*

In the UK death certified by brain-based criteria is defined as the 'irreversible loss of the capacity for consciousness combined with the irreversible loss of the capacity to breathe' (Working Group 1995: 381). This diagnosis needs to be established clinically with certain pre-conditions that must be met and specific exclusions that must be verified; finally the function of the brain must be established by clinical tests. The pre-conditions and exclusions that are required to establish brainstem death in adults in the UK are listed in Box 5.1. The clinical tests used for the confirmation of brainstem death are listed in Box 5.2.

Box 5.1 UK criteria for the diagnosis of death using brainstem testing in adults (Department of Health 1998)

Three steps need to be carried out so that a diagnosis of brainstem death can be made and they are:

That certain **(1) preconditions** have been met, these are: (i) there should be no doubt that the patient's condition is due to irremediable brain damage of known aetiology and (ii) that the patient is deeply unconscious on a ventilator.

That the above preconditions are not due to any reversible causes of apnoeic coma, so certain **(2) exclusions** must be met and they are: (i) that there should be no evidence that this state is due to depressant drugs, (ii) that primary hypothermia as a cause of unconsciousness has been excluded (temperature is greater than <35° C), that (iii) potentially reversible circulatory, metabolic and endocrine disturbances have been excluded as a cause of continuing unconsciousness, and finally that on (3) **clinical testing** (see Box 5.2) all brainstem reflexes are absent and the patient is apnoeic.

Box 5.2 Clinical tests for the diagnosis of death based on brainstem criteria (Department of Health 1998)

The following brainstem reflexes are then tested systematically (Pallis and Harley 1996) as the clinician is seeking:

- No pupillary response to light.
- No corneal reflex when the cornea is stimulated.
- No vestibule-ocular reflex during the slow injection of at least 50mls of ice-cold water over 1 minute into each external auditory canal in turn.
- No motor response within the cranial nerve distribution during adequate stimulation of any somatic area.
- No limb response to supraorbital pressure or as Pallis and Harley (1996) state 'there should be no grimacing in response to painful stimuli applied either to the trigeminal fields (firm supraorbital pressure) or to the limbs'.
- No gag reflex or reflex response to bronchial stimulation by suction catheter placed down the trachea.
- No respiratory movements occur when the patient is disconnected from the mechanical ventilator. The aim of this test is for the arterial carbon dioxide to exceed the levels that would stimulate respiration, so the $PaCO_2$ should reach 6.65KPa (50mm Hg).

To prevent hypoxia the patient should be pre-oxygenated with 100% oxygen delivered at 6 litres per minute for 10 minutes, then ventilated with 5% CO_2 in oxygen for 5 minutes. The ventilator should then be disconnected for 10 minutes while100% oxygen is delivered at 6 litres per minute via a catheter inserted into the trachea which reaches the carina.

The diagnosis of brainstem death

The diagnosis of brainstem death is presented to families who are faced with the reality of a body that is warm and pink, that has a pulse and a chest that rises and falls. It is therefore not surprising that understanding death as certified by brainstem testing is an important factor in families' decision-making (Pearson *et al.* 1995; Franz *et al.* 1997) and also an issue that has been shown to impact on subsequent grief (Burroughs *et al.* 1998; Sque *et al.* 2003). Despite this issue being an important one, studies carried out with donating and non-donating family members report poor understanding of the meaning of brain death (Pearson *et al.* 1995; DeJong *et al.* 1998; Beaulieu 1999; Siminoff *et al.* 2003), dissatisfaction with the quality and method of information-sharing regarding brain death (Pearson *et al.* 1995), dissatisfaction with the decision made at request (Burroughs *et al.* 1998) and confusion with other neurological conditions, for example, coma and the persistent vegetative state (PVS) (Franz *et al.* 1997).

Pelletier (1993: 153), who interviewed donating family members only, reported, respondents receiving 'minimal, if any, information about the diagnosis of brain death', while Haddow (2004) found that a majority of participants in her study were unaware of the procedures (tests) that would be carried out to establish brainstem death. While studies have also reported satisfaction with the amount and type of information offered to respondents regarding brain death (Douglass and Daly 1995; Franz *et al.* 1997; Haddow 2004), when Franz *et al.* asked participants specific questions to assess their knowledge regarding the diagnosis they found that despite saying that they were satisfied with the type and amount of information regarding brain death there was poor understanding of this diagnosis and confusion between brain death and other neurological states. Six years later, Siminoff *et al.* (2003) reported that while nearly all the families in their research (96 per cent of 403 families of organ donor eligible patients) had been told that their family member was brain dead, only 28 per cent of their sample were able to provide a correct definition of brain death when asked by researchers.

A further issue is that the diagnosis of death by brainstem testing may be confounded by the terminology used by health professionals in relation to the care of critically injured patients. Language such as 'being kept alive on the ventilator', and 'life support' colludes to undermine the message that death is inevitable (or has already occurred). Franz *et al.* (1997) goes so far as to say that the term life-support should *never* be used in relation to the care of the brain dead patient due to the possibility of confusion regarding death. The term brainstem death may itself suggest that death certified by brainstem testing is inclusive to the brain and exclusive of the body. This choice of language may undermine the acceptance of the irreversibility of the brain injury sustained and may support the view that the family member could recover with intensive rehabilitation.

It would appear that information regarding death diagnosed by brainstem testing is, generally, not well delivered and poorly understood, and in view of this asking family members if they would like to attend and observe testing may be an option worth considering. Sque *et al.* (2003) reported that four family members indicated that they were asked if they wanted to be present and observe brainstem testing and while these participants were apprehensive, they reported that observing the tests confirmed what the medical staff had told them (see Box 5.3). Sque *et al.* also reported that family members who chose not to be present at testing felt that the offer of this opportunity showed a desire by the staff to involve them in what was happening to their relative and to keep them fully informed.

Box 5.3 A personal experience of brainstem testing

Around four o'clock the consultant anaesthetist Dr R came and he was going to do the second lot of tests, and we were present while he did them. He said that he'd never done it with relatives present before. He explained it all in beautiful, simple language for my daughter J and didn't patronize or make her feel out of it because she was the only non-medical person in the room. I was glad that he let us stay. He did ask us did we want to leave? And I was glad because I felt J in particular didn't believe it. She kept saying I haven't finished with him yet, I haven't finished with him yet. I was glad because it meant that she would actually be sure, and I knew that I wanted them to be sure that there wasn't any hope at all, because I imagine that as we went through the process towards him going up to theatre that there'd be a lot of uncertainty. Was he really, was he really dead? I was really glad and grateful for that opportunity for them, particularly J. M has seen far more of it than I have, and I imagined she wouldn't have any doubts, but for J it would be much better like that. And Dr R was extremely gentle, extremely careful, used really helpful language and he also warned us that it would be a very long drawn out thing. He gave us a reasonable accurate picture of how long it would take for everything to happen.
(S34721, 36210)

There is evidence that some units in the UK are offering the opportunity of observing brainstem testing to family members. Pugh *et al.* (2000) report that 32 per cent of consultants and 42 per cent of senior nurses that they contacted had experience of a relative's presence during testing and that 69 per cent of those contacted felt that it was helpful for relatives. Forty-five per cent of these health professionals said they would be more willing to allow the next of kin to view brainstem testing if there was adequate support in the form of a dedicated person to support families and to carry out careful explanations related to problems such as spinal reflexes.[2]

The provision of a videotape or DVD demonstrating the procedure of brainstem testing, which could be viewed by family members and health care professionals is also an option. The provision of such a visual aid may provide a medium through which questions regarding death and brainstem testing could be answered as well as offering an opportunity to discredit images related to coma that are often attributed to brainstem death such as, *'Well I heard you can wake up after two years in a coma'*. Franz *et al.* (1997: 20) support the production of a video that is viewed with a health professional in attendance, as in their view 'a pre-recorded message means that the information [about brain death] could be organized and presented in a clear, concise, and reliable way with the videotape concentrating on conveying basic facts about brain death, the team member could focus on answering the family's questions and attending to their emotional needs'.

It is clear from the work by Sque *et al.* (2003) that family members who watched brainstem testing were seeking confirmation of death and the fact that some family members were still unclear about what brainstem tests were, and how these tests related to the death of their family member, at two years post bereavement, is testimony to the need for change in practice in this area. The sheer load and complexity of information that is presented, and then added to, if families agree to organ donation, is immense. Therefore better information-sharing techniques are required, methods that can work together to enhance the understanding and retention of complicated information such as brain injury, brain anatomy and brainstem testing. While the type and method of information-sharing in hospital is only one of the factors that influence donation decisions, it may be that it is a far more influential factor than had been previously considered.

The need for information

The need for accurate, understandable and consistent information regarding the illness trajectory in relation to organ donation has been reported by other authors (Pelletier 1993; Pearson *et al.* 1995; Franz *et al.* 1997; Sque 2001; Sque *et al.* 2005; Long *et al.* 2006) and has been shown to be the most commonly identified need for family members in the intensive care unit (ICU) (Hickey and Leske 1992; Lorenz 1995; Zazpe *et al.* 1997). Fulfilling the informational needs of family members has been shown to reduce anxiety, especially if more than one channel of communication is used to transmit the desired information (Zazpe *et al.* 1997), and yet it has been reported as one of the most poorly met needs within the ICU (Barbret *et al.* 1997). A number of factors would appear to be relevant to this poorly met need and they include: the methods used to transmit information; the content of the information; the state of mind of the person receiving the information; the nature of the critical injury and diagnosis of death; and the skills of health professionals in sharing knowledge. How can information-sharing techniques meet the needs of the family members of a potential organ donor?

Information-sharing

In relation to the means by which information is shared, most institutions use, predominantly, one channel of communication, verbal communication, to deliver information to family members. For example, complicated information such as that regarding the nature of brain injury is often given without an assessment of family members' prior knowledge of brain anatomy or function, a situation which Sque *et al.* (2003) report may leave family members struggling to understand what the injury means in relation to the quality of life of their family member. Sque *et al.* and Pearson *et al.* (1995) suggest that family members can be assisted in understanding the nature and severity of brain injury when more 'visual' means of information-sharing are used, as shown in Table 5.1.

Table 5.1 Methods used to increase understanding of the critical brain injury

Method	How method was perceived to help
Talking	Responsive
Seeing CT scans	Confirmatory
Seeing X-rays	Illustrative
Use of anatomical models	Explanatory
Witnessing brainstem testing	Confirmatory
Reading and sharing information leaflets	Informative and stimulating discussion

Sque *et al.* (2003) reported that the understanding of family members in relation to the injury sustained by their relative was more detailed in those who had been exposed to one or more of the methods listed in Table 5.1. Added to this, the authors report that family members who had experienced these methods of communicating information had fewer questions about the nature of the injury at two years post-bereavement. The methods listed in Table 5.1 are reported to help families in specific ways as indicated by the following comments:

- Being shown CT scans and x-rays and having the critical injury explained. 'He showed us the brain scan which was just amazing, all this black (bleeding).' (t5322,5488)
- The use of an anatomical model of the brain to indicate the area of the injury, the damage caused and the consequences of the damage. 'He brought in a model of the brain with removable bits which he took apart and showed us which bit was affected. That really put us in the picture.' (t/tbhfieldnotes)

- Being present when brainstem testing was carried out. 'Yes. He [doctor] was absolutely brilliant. He said he had one set of tests and they had done the scan which showed that there wasn't anything that could be done, and so after a period of time, I don't know how long it was, hours, he was going to do another set of tests. And he said we could be in there to see them if we wanted to or not. And I think we were probably the only people who ever said we wanted to be there. But from their point of view I think, I wanted to see what they were doing to him and I wanted to be sure that he really was dead.' (s/m12699,13235)

There appeared to be added benefits to using methods such as those listed in Table 5.1, as family members in the Sque *et al.* (2003) study reported feeling: that staff had 'included them in a meaningful way in what was happening', and that they felt 'fully informed' and 'involved'. Although studies have reported the expressed wish of family members in ICU to have methods such as X-rays, diagrams, models or pictures used to explain the patient's brain injury (Pearson *et al.* 1995; Franz *et al.* 1997; Sque *et al.* 2005) these options are not regularly used by health professionals. In the USA, Franz *et al.* (1997) reported that informational aids such as *The Brain Injured Patient Flipchart* (Boschert *et al.* 1991) and *The Injured Brain* (Youngstein and Davis 1993) are available, but that there is only limited use of such aids. Not only are the methods used for communicating information a factor in facilitating families in understanding what is happening to their relative, but the context of the information being communicated may impair their ability to process what they are being told or shown, due to emotions such as shock, anger, disbelief and sadness. These emotions appear to create a particular emotional landscape within which the family member must make complex decisions and can be a barrier to processing the information being shared with them by the nursing and medical teams.

Barriers to information-sharing

Interview data from the Sque *et al.* (2003) study indicated how much time family members spent in a form of 'internal dialogue'. This involved 'recalling' the deceased and the life spent together, the last conversation with the deceased, 'hoping' that the family member would survive and, for some, bargaining with God. These dialogues or ruminations acted as 'pull factors', drawing the family member away from the informational flow around them. As the time in hospital extended the internal dialogue and ruminations changed and were influenced by 'push factors', such as thoughts of brain damage and death, which focused family members toward the informational flow available to them and triggered some to become extra vigilant of monitoring equipment and to seek *repeated reassurances'* from medical and nursing staff. The nature of this emotional landscape is well described in Chapter 4 as the theory of dissonant loss (Sque and Payne 1996).

In view of this internal dialogue about the deceased, and its potential impact as a barrier to information-sharing it is essential that health professionals gain the attention of the specific next of kin and establish what participants referred to as 'rapport'.

Overcoming barriers to information sharing

A positive rapport between the family and the health care team appears to facilitate communication and discussions about the diagnosis of death, and the request for organ and tissue donation. Rapport resulted from an assessment by the family member regarding the care that they and other relatives received during the time in hospital. Care that acknowledged the needs of the next of kin, in relation to understanding what was happening to their family member, and acknowledged them as the important person in the patient's life was a particular feature of rapport. A husband explains:

> He was excellent. And what he did, he brought the scans in and put them up on the window. He didn't talk to the other people he spoke to me. And him and I, like he explained everything to me and he answered my questions and whatever, and he was very good. (s/r23899,24049)

The quality of care demonstrated by health professionals and the resulting rapport appeared to leave lasting positive memories. While Pearson *et al.* (1995) did not find an association between hospital treatment and the decision to donate, DeJong *et al.* (1998) indicate that there is an association between the perceived quality of care for the dying or deceased and a positive donation decision. Sque *et al.* (2003) also found a link between the quality of care experienced and the decision to donate, while Haddow (2004) reports the influence of 'a bond of trust' on decision-making.

Research (Pearson *et al.* 1995; DeJong *et al.* 1998; Sque *et al.* 2003, 2005; Haddow 2004) indicates that for families to feel supported in their decision-making regarding organ donation, family members need, *time* – to understand and absorb the nature of the brain injury which had killed their family member so suddenly, and to discuss this with other family members and seek reassurances for any concerns; *attention* – to the special role that they hold as next of kin, to their inner turmoil and the understanding that this could impact on how they process information; and *care* – in the way, and the where, that information is presented and the understanding that this will 'live' on in their minds for years to come (see Figure 5.1).

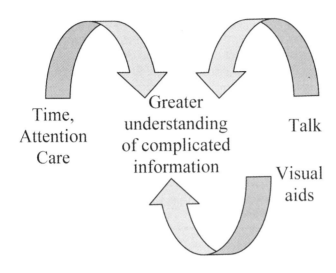

Time,
Attention
Care

Greater
understanding
of complicated
information

Talk

Visual
aids

Figure 5.1 Multiple methods of communicating information underpinned by time, attention and care leads to greater understanding of complicated information

Barriers to discussing organ donation

Health professionals are the 'gatekeepers' to the donation process and this can be problematic as some hesitate in making a request, feeling that discussing donation is intrusive in the family's moment of grief (Kiberd and Kiberd 1992; Kent 2002), others are disinterested in, or discomforted by, organ donation (Daneffel *et al.* 1992), upset by the circumstances surrounding organ donation or the donation operation (Pallis and Harley 1996) or are not positive about organ donation (Siminoff and Miller 1994; Sque *et al.* 2000). While health professionals may feel reluctant to raise the issue of organ donation with family members there is evidence to support the view that many family members do not have an objection to organ donation being discussed with them (Randhawa 1995; Sque *et al.* 2003). Furthermore, Sque *et al.* (2003) reported that none of the family members in their study, including those who declined organ donation, felt that they should not have been asked, or that the discussion about organ donation increased their distress levels as '*The worst thing that could have happened already had*' – i.e. the death of their family member. Pelletier (1993) goes so far as to say that donating family members *needed* health professionals to ask them about organ donation, needed them to respond to their request to donate (if the next of kin raised the issue first) and to discuss what organs and tissues could be donated.

There is no doubt that some family members will be shocked, surprised or distressed at being approached about organ donation, as reported by Pearson *et al.* (1995) but it is important to bear in mind the impact of sudden death, and the influence that this may have. Sudden death not only robs the next of kin of a significant relationship without warning, but also robs them of many of their usual coping mechanisms imposing a sequence of events that leaves them feeling dispossessed of physical and psychological equilibrium. It is therefore not surprising that some family members decline donation, or that some are angry at being asked to consider organ donation. In these situations the person making the approach may choose to 'back off' in the face of dissent. There is a risk here however that the person who protests most loudly may not be the person who will suffer the greatest consequences from a decision made at this time, a decision that may be regretted later due to a lack of discussion regarding their views.

The needs of the next of kin, or the person whom the deceased would expect to make decisions on their behalf, must be elicited even in the face of another family member who is forthright and demanding. Those making an approach to families may need to speak to any 'forthright' person and discuss with them the possible consequences of a decision that may be regretted later because of the disproportionate influence of their views. Health professionals involved in requesting should be prepared to investigate through questioning (DeJong *et al.* 1998; Verble and Worth 1999, 2000), relatives' views regarding organ donation, as it is a once in a lifetime decision, which once made cannot be unmade.[3]

Sque *et al.* (2003) and Randhawa (1995) found that families did not feel that being asked about organ donation increased their distress, or that organ donation should not have been raised by the health care team. However, it is important that the families' distress, anger or emotional outbursts, caused by the suddenness of the death, are not misinterpreted and allowed to become a barrier to facilitating decisions that may impact adversely on bereavement. Families need every opportunity to reach a decision that will remain right for them and this can be facilitated further by health professionals gaining specific education in relation to individual differences, belief systems, stress reactions and how these issues can be addressed through communication skills training.

Factors influencing the donation decision

Knowing the wishes of the deceased in relation to organ donation is the most important influence on family members' decision-making (Douglass and Daly 1995; Pearson *et al.* 1995; Sque and Payne 1996; DeJong *et al.* 1998; Martinez *et al.* 2001; Sque *et al.* 2003; Haddow 2004) and has been reported as a predictor of organ donation (Burroughs *et al.* 1998). Next of kin who know the wishes of the deceased regarding organ donation usually, but not always (Sque *et al.* 2006), make decisions in line with those wishes.

Family members may have 'concrete knowledge' of the wishes of the deceased in the form of organ donor cards or passports which had been signed, or 'discursive knowledge' (Sque *et al.* 2003) whereby the family member had discussed their wishes regarding organ donation.

The discussion about an individual's wish regarding organ donation has been cited as having particular importance if family members are to feel assured in their decision-making. Burroughs *et al.* (1998) reported that in the situation where an organ donor card had been signed and no discussion had taken place, that family members were less assured in their decision-making. So the combination of a signed card and a personal discussion appeared to increase the confidence with which family members made decisions about donation.

In cases where family members initiate discussions about donation the following factors have been highlighted as influencing their approach to health professionals: knowing the views of the deceased; being concerned that the family would not be asked; wanting to ensure that the staff knew the wishes of the deceased; and being concerned about the impact on the health professionals of asking the family about organ donation and wanting to ameliorate this effect (Sque *et al.* 2003).

A decision to donate, when the views of the deceased were not known, was influenced by the perceived 'attributes' of the deceased and the view of them held by next of kin and extended family as an 'altruistic person' who 'cared for others' and who 'was always doing things for others'. In this situation the deceased was also understood to have a neutral stance regarding organ donation. Family members were also motivated to donate by a need to help others (in line with the lifestyle of the deceased) and the need for something positive to come out of the negative experience of this sudden death (Sque *et al.* 2003, 2005).

A decision to decline donation has been linked to: the deceased's opposition to donation and/or not knowing the wishes of the deceased (Douglass and Daly 1995; Pearson *et al.* 1995; DeJong *et al.* 1998; Martinez *et al.* 2001; Sque *et al.* 2003, 2005; Haddow 2004); dissatisfaction with the care provided to the deceased and/or the family (DeJong *et al.* 1998; Rosel *et al.* 1999);

religious, personal and cultural beliefs (Radecki and Jaccard 1997; Burroughs *et al.* 1998; Rodrique *et al.* 2004; Crowley-Matoka and Lock 2006); lack of trust in the health care services (Haustein and Sellers 2004; Sanner 2006); and beliefs that health care professionals will not strive to save a person if they are aware that they have agreed to be an organ donor (Riether and Mahler 1995; Sanner 2006), among other factors.

Although religious beliefs have been listed as being a barrier to organ donation, according to the speakers representing Judaism, Buddhism, Islam, Catholicism, Sikhism and Christianity who presented their perspective at an interfaith symposium (the Organ Donation Conference, Wednesday 10 September 2003, convened by UK Transplant and the Church of England Hospital Chaplaincies Council), none of these religions disagree with the giving of an organ to save a life. Most religions either support organ donation or leave the decision to the discretion of the individual.[4] What appears to be the barrier are cultural beliefs related to the treatment of the body at and after death, and the possible need for an intact body in the afterlife (Riether and Mahler 1995; Crowley-Matoka and Lock 2006). The following example is offered to demonstrate the interplay of religious and cultural beliefs.

Japan has a rich religious heritage drawing influences from the Shinto, Taoist, Confucian and Buddhist traditions (Craven and Rodin 1992). Some authors suggest that it is the combination of beliefs from these religions that underpin the Japanese discomfort with the concept of brain death and the Japanese government's decision to support the diagnosis of brain death only for those who wish their organs to be donated and who have documented this wish, and have gained the support of their family (Craven and Rodin 1992; McConnell 1999; Lock 2002). Harmonization with nature is one of the three basic goals of Shinto and while the Shinto faith accepts removal of bodily organs if it is for the saving of a life, Shinto followers also believe that declaring death before the heart stops is against nature. In relation to Confucianism, Taoism and Buddhism, it is the role of the afterlife that is a barrier to organ donation as there is a need for the body to be whole. These beliefs have led to a social consensus in Japan that sees transplantation as devaluing life, and the afterlife (McConnell 1999).

The ability to interchange human organs and tissues introduces a spectrum of need that can only be fulfilled by a clear understanding of how critical injury, sudden death and the diagnosis of death by brainstem testing can impact on family members' decision-making regarding organ donation. Assessment of informational needs should begin at the bedside with emergency care and ICU health professionals assessing families' immediate needs for information, contact with their injured relative, the type of support they have available, their emotional response to what is happening, and their personal and cultural beliefs regarding the appropriate treatment of the body at and after death. This assessment can be shared with other health professionals, for example transplant coordinators and bereavement support workers so that they can continue to support families during their bereavement.

Conclusion

This chapter has discussed some of the factors that impact on family members who experience the sudden death of a relative, and who after that person is diagnosed dead using neurological criteria are approached about donating organs, focusing on a number of studies from the last 15 years of research. The issues discussed that could be addressed in the clinical environment are:

- assessment of individual informational needs, available support and emotional responses to the ongoing situation;
- the development and use of visual information aids (e.g. a video that explains the nature of brain injury and death certified by brainstem testing);
- the offer of the opportunity for family members to attend brainstem testing if they wish to do so;
- identification of, and acknowledgement of, the person who the deceased would expect to make decisions about them (this may not be the legal next of kin);[5]
- the discussion about organ donation should be carried out by, and restricted to, those staff members who are comfortable with and knowledgeable about this topic;
- a discussion regarding the donation decision should be carried out to reduce the possibility of a decision that may be regretted later;
- education of all health professionals regarding the bereavement needs of families whose family member has died suddenly with specific attention to individual differences, belief systems, stress reactions and therapeutic questioning techniques.

By addressing these issues families can be supported in making decisions about organ donation that they are confident in and remain comfortable with throughout their subsequent bereavement.

Notes

1   Presently in the UK 'death certified by brainstem testing' is preferred to the term 'brainstem death'.
2   Spinal reflexes can result in involuntary movements, or jerks of the limbs that can cause family members to doubt the diagnosis of death.

3   It is our understanding that transplant coordinators are encouraged to carry out 'gentle questioning' in relation to reasons why the family/individual does not want to proceed with organ donation. Gentle questioning may not be carried out when a transplant coordinator is not involved in the donation discussion. This questioning will help clarify views held by the family and the deceased. Encouraging the family to articulate their views would indicate the strength with which these views are held.

4   For details of other religions or belief groups see the webpage of Transplant for Life at www.transsplantsforlife.org/miracles/religions.html.

5   In the UK Human Tissue Act (2004) states in Part 1, Section 2 that in the case of a child 'appropriate consent means the consent of a person who has parental responsibility for him [the child]'. Section 3 states that in the case of an adult 'appropriate consent' rests with 'a nominated person' or 'person who stood in a qualifying relationship to him immediately before he died'. This person may not necessarily be the next of kin. There are a number of criteria given defining a nominated person and a qualifying relationship.

References

Ad Hoc Committee of the Harvard Medical School (1968) A definition of irreversible coma, *Journal of the American Medical Journal*, 205(6): 337–40.

Barbret, L.C., Westphal, C.G. and Daly, G.A. (1997) Meeting the informational needs of families of critical care patients, *Journal of Healthcare Quality*, 9(2): 5–9.

Beaulieu, D. (1999) Organ donation: the family's right to make an informed choice, *Journal of Neuroscience Nursing*, 31(1): 37–42.

Boschert, A., Reed, E. and Worth, D. (1991) *The Brain Injured Patient Flipchart*. Louisville, KY: Kentucky Organ Donor Affiliates.

Burroughs, T.E., Hong, B.A., Kappel, D.F. and Freedman, B.K. (1998) The stability of family decisions to consent or refuse organ donation. Would you do it again? *Psychosomatic Medicine*, 60: 156–62.

Capron, A.M. (1999) The bifurcated legal standard for determining death, in S.J. Youngner, R.M. Arnold and R. Schapiro (eds) *The Definition of Death: Contemporary Controversies*. Baltimore, MD: Johns Hopkins University Press.

Craven, J. and Rodin, G.M. (1992) *Psychiatric Aspects of Organ Transplantation*. Oxford: Oxford University Press.

Crowley-Matoka, M. and Lock, M. (2006) Organ transplantation in a globalized world, *Mortality*, 11(2): 166–81.

Danneffel, M.B., Kappes, J.E., Waltmire II, D. and Yearwood, L. (1992) Knowledge and attitudes of health care professionals about organ and tissue donation, *Journal of Transplant Coordination*, 2(3): 2531–2.

DeJong, W., Franz, H.G., Wolfe, S.M., Nathan, H., Payne, D., Reitsma, W. and Beasley, C. (1998) Requesting organ donation: an interview study of donor and non-donor families, *American Journal of Critical Care*, 7: 13–23.

Department of Health and Social Security Report of the Working Party (1983) *Cadaveric Organs for Transplantation: A Code of Practice Including the Diagnosis of Brain Death*. London: HMSO.

Department of Health (1998) *A Code of Practice for the Diagnosis of Brain Stem Death: Including Guidelines for the Identification and Management of Potential Organ and Tissue Donors*. London: Department of Health.

Douglass, G.E. and Daly, M. (1995) Donor families' experience of organ donation, *Anaesthesia and Intensive Care*, 23(1): 96–8.

Evans, M. and Potts, M. (2000) Narrative case against brain death, in M. Potts, P.A. Byrne and R.G. Nilges (eds) *Beyond Brain Death: The Case Against Brain Based Criteria for Human Death*. London: Kluwer Academic Publishers.

Franz, H.G., DeJong, W., Wolfe, S.M., Nathan, H., Payne, D., Reitsma, W. and Beasley, C. (1997) Explaining brain death: a critical feature of the donation process, *Journal of Transplant Coordination*, 7: 14–21.

Haddow, G. (2004) Donor and nondonor families' accounts of communication and relations with health care professionals, *Progress in Transplantation*, 14(1): 41–8.

Haupt, W.F. and Rudolf, J. (1999) European brain death codes: a comparison of national guidelines, *Journal of Neurology*, 246(6): 432–7.

Haustein, S. and Sellers, M.T. (2004) Factors associated with (un)willingness to an organ donor: importance of public exposure and knowledge, *Clinical Transplantation*, 18: 193–200.

Hickey, M.L. and Leske, J.S. (1992) Needs of families of critically ill patients: state of the science and future directions, *Critical Care Nurse*, 4(4): 645–9.

Kent, B. (2002) Psychosocial factors influencing nurses' involvement with organ and tissue donation, *International Journal of Nursing Studies*, 39: 429–40.

Kiberd, M.C. and Kiberd, B.A. (1992) Nursing attitudes towards organ donation, procurement, and transplantation, *Heart and Lung*, 21(2): 106–11.

Lock, M. (2002) *Twice Dead: Organ Transplants and the Reinvention of Death*. Berkeley, CA: University of California Press.

Long, T., Sque, M. and Payne, S. (2006) Information sharing: its impact on donor and non-donor families' experiences in hospital, *Progress in Transplantation*, 16(2): 144–9.

Lorenz, B.T. (1995) Needs of family members of critically ill adults, *MEDSURG Nursing*, 4(6): 445–51.

Martinez, J.M., Lopez, J.S., Martin, A., Martin, M.J., Scandroglio, B. and Martin, J.M. (2001) Organ donation and family decision-making within the Spanish system, *Social Science & Medicine*, 53: 405–21.

McConnell, J.R. (1999) The ambiguity about death in Japan: an ethical implication for organ procurement, *Journal of Medical Ethics*, 25: 322–4.

Mollaret, P. And Goulon, M. (1959) La coma depass, *Revue Neurologique*, 101: 3–15.

Pallis, C. (1994) Brain stem death: the evolution of a concept, in P.J. Morris (ed.) *Kidney Transplantation: Principles and Practice*, 4th edn. London: W.B. Saunders.

Pallis, C. and Harley, D.H. (1996) *ABC of Brainstem Death*. London: British Medical Publications.

Pearson, I.Y., Bazeley, P., Spencer-Plane, T., Chapman, J.R. and Robertson, P. (1995) A survey of families of brain dead patients: their experiences, attitudes to organ donation and transplantation, *Anaesthesia and Intensive Care*, 23(1): 88–95.

Pelletier, M. (1993) The needs of family members of organ and tissue donors, *Heart and Lung*, 22(2): 151–7.

Powner, D.J. and Darby, J.M. (1999) Current considerations in the issue of brain death, *Neurosurgery*, 45(5): 1222–6.

President's Commission for the Study of Ethical Problems in Medicine and Biomedical and Behavioral Research (1981) *Defining Death: Medical, Legal and Ethical Issues in the Definition of Death*. Washington, DC: US Congress.

Pugh, J., Clarke, L., Gray, J., Haveman, J., Lawler, P. and Nonner, S. (2000) Presence of relatives during testing of brain stem death: questionnaire study, *British Medical Journal*, 321: 1505–6.

Radecki, C.M. and Jaccard, J. (1997) Psychological aspects of organ donation: a critical review and synthesis of individual and next-of-kin donation decisions, *Health Psychology*, 6(2): 183–95.

Rawdhawa, G. (1995) Organ donation: social and cultural issues, *Nursing Standard*, 9(41): 25–7.

Riether, A.M. and Mahler, E. (1995) Organ donation: psychiatric, social, and ethical considerations, *Psychosomatics*, 36(4): 336–43.

Rodrique, J.R., Cornell, D.L., Jackson, S.I., Danasky, W., Marhefka, S. and Reed, A.I. (2004) Are organ donation attitudes and beliefs, empathy, and life orientation related to donor registration status? *Progress in Transplantation*, 14(1): 56–60.

Rosel, J., Frutos, M.A., Blanca, M.J. and Ruiz, P. (1999) Discriminant variables between organ donors and nondonors: a post hoc investigation, *Journal of Transplant Coordination*, 9(1): 50–3.

Sanner, M. (2006) People's attitudes and reactions to organ donation, *Mortality*, 11(2): 133–50.

Saunders, C.M. (1993) Risk factors in bereavement, in M. Stroebe, W. Stroebe and R.O. Hansson (eds) *Handbook of Bereavement: Theory, Research and Intervention*. Cambridge: Cambridge University Press.

Siminoff, L.A. and Miller, A.R. (1994) Differences in the procurement of organs and tissues by health care professionals, *Clinical Transplantation*, 8(5): 460–5.

Siminoff, L.A., Mercer, L.A. and Arnold, R. (2003) Families' understanding of brain death, *Progress in Transplantation*, 13(3): 218–24.

Sque, M. (2001) Being a carer in acute crisis: the situation for relatives of organ donors, in S. Payne and C. Ellis-Hill (eds) *Chronic and Terminal Illness: New Perspectives on Caring and Carers*. Oxford: Oxford University Press.

Sque, M. and Payne, S. (1996) Dissonant loss: the experiences of donor relatives, *Social Science & Medicine*, 43(9): 1359–70.

Sque, M., Payne, S. and Vlachonikolis, I. (2000) Cadaveric donotransplantation: nurses' attitudes, knowledge and behaviour, *Social Science and Medicine*, 50: 541–52.

Sque, M., Long, T. and Payne, S. (2003) *Organ and Tissue Donation: Exploring the Needs of Families*. Final report of a three-year study commissioned by the British Organ Donor Society, funded by the Community Fund. University of Southampton, Southampton: UK.

Sque, M., Long, T. and Payne, S. (2005) Organ donation: key factors influencing families' decision-making, *Transplantation Proceedings*, 37: 543–6.

Sque, M., Long, T., Payne, S. and Allardyce, D. (2006) *Exploring the End of Life Decision-making and Hospital Experiences of Families Who Did Not Donate Organs for Transplant Operations*. Final Research Report for UK Transplant. University of Southampton, Southampton: UK.

Tilney, N.L. (2003) *Transplantation: From Myth to Reality*. New Haven, CT: Yale University Press.

Verble, M. and Worth, J. (1999) Dealing with the fear of mutilation in the donation discussion, *Journal of Transplant Coordination*, 9: 54–6.

Verble, M. and Worth, J. (2000) Fears and concerns expressed by families in the donation discussion, *Progress in Transplantation*, 10(1): 48–53.

Wertheimer, P., Jouvet, M. and Descotes, J. (1959) A respiration artificielle propos du diagnostic de la mort du systeme nerveux dans les comas aces arrêt respiratoire traites par la, *Presse Médicine*, 67: 87–8.

Working Group of Conferences of Royal Medical Colleges and Their Faculties in the United Kingdom (1976) Diagnosis of death, *British Medical Journal*, 2: 1187–8.

Working Group convened by the Royal College of Physicians and Endorsed by the Conference of Medical Royal Colleges and Their Faculties in the United Kingdom (1995) Criteria for the diagnosis of brain stem death, *Journal of the Royal College of Physicians*, 29(5): 381–2.

Wright, B. (1996) *Sudden Death: A Research Base for Practice*, 2nd edn. New York: Churchill Livingstone.

Youngstein, K.P. and Davis, F.D. (1993) *The Injured Brain*. New York: Biocom.

Zazpe, C., Margall, M.A., Otano, C., Perochena, M.P. and Asiain, M.C. (1997) Meeting needs of family members of critically ill patients in a Spanish intensive care unit, *Intensive Critical Care Nursing*, 13(1): 12–16.

6 Tissue donation and the attitudes of health care professionals

Bridie Kent

Introduction

Since the first corneal transplant in 1905, improved surgical techniques and the development of immunosuppressive drugs have led to excellent success rates for organ and tissue transplantation procedures. This chapter will focus on the cadaveric donation of tissue and the attitudes towards it of health professionals, because they are key players in the donation-transplantation process.

The chapter begins with an overview of cadaveric tissue donation, including what can currently be transplanted. It will then present what is known about health professionals' attitudes to and knowledge of tissue donation and the impact that these have on donation rates. Attitudes, their components and their effect upon behaviour are explored using theories arising from social psychology to explain how these influence actual or intended behaviours associated with the discussion of donation wishes with relatives of the potential donor. Since some tissues, such as blood and bone marrow, can only normally be donated during life, these will be excluded since the behaviours associated with blood donation differ significantly from those associated with cadaveric tissue donation.

Tissue donation

Before progressing further, it is timely to explain what tissue can be donated and why tissue donation and transplantation are differentiated from that of organs, because, arguably, all the material transplanted is human tissue. It is generally accepted that organ donation and transplantation refers to solid organs such as heart, lung, liver and kidney. Tissue, however, includes the following:

- corneas, sclera, and other optical material;
- bone;
- skin;
- heart valves.

In the past 20 years, composite tissue allotransplantation has advanced significantly, with the first successful hand transplant carried out in 1998 (Kann *et al.* 2000) and recently a face transplant has been undertaken in France (Devauchelle *et al.* 2006). Such tissue transplants mark a new phase in reconstructive surgery undertaken to repair the face, larynx and extremities (Cunningham *et al.* 2004) and will present health professionals and the public with yet more challenges to add to those already posed by the established types of tissue donation.

The key difference between organ and tissue donation is that organs are dependent on a functioning blood supply because without this the organs deteriorate rapidly and are unsuitable for subsequent transplantation. Tissue, on the other hand, is retrieved when the heart is no longer beating, and this generally takes place several hours or longer after asystolic death has been confirmed. Since tissue is transplanted in an avascular state, the quality of the match between donor and recipient that is vital for the success of organ transplantation is less of an issue.

Table 6.1 summarizes the retrieval maximums and other criteria for the main tissues donated after death required by the British Association of Tissue Banking (www.batb.org.uk/).

The numbers of potential tissue donors worldwide are much greater than for organ donation, due primarily to the circumstances of the death. Corneal and other tissue can be donated not only by those who have suffered brain death, but also from those who have died from asystole (non-heartbeating donors). It is estimated that only 1.5 to 3 per cent of the population in the western world die in the circumstances of brain death, cared for in the intensive care unit, while for more than half of all hospital deaths corneal donation is a possibility (Metropolitan Health and Aged Services Division 2004). Persons who have died at home, in hospices, rest homes, community hospitals, as well as those who die in acute care settings can all be perceived as potential tissue donors.

Tissues are often transplanted into the recipient days or weeks after the donation has taken place. Most are stored in tissue banks after infection clearance has been given. Bone, for example, is stripped of anything not required, cleaned thoroughly and then sterilized before storage. Corneas are separated from the eye (which may be removed intact at the time of donation), inspected for quality and then stored in a protective medium for 30 days until infection clearance has been given and then 'banked' in what are, in reality, large refrigerators. Heart valves are also inspected and cleaned prior

Table 6.1 Tissue donor acceptance criteria

Tissue	Heart valves	Corneas	Skin	Bone	Tendons
Age limit (years)	0–60	>3	17–75	17–75	18–45
Time limit after death (hours)	48	24	24	24	24
Uses	• Save the lives of children born with severely deformed hearts • Save or improve the lives of adults with diseased or infected valves	• Restore sight in patients with diseased or opaque corneas • Scleral tissue is used for reconstructive surgery	• Skin grafts can act as temporary or permanent biological covering	• Used in a variety of orthopaedic procedures to reduce patients' pain and restore their mobility	• Are transplanted to restore mobility and stability in knee joints

Used with permission of the British Association for Tissue Banking.

to storage in heart valve banks. Skin is removed from the cadaver using a specially designed tool, to generate very thin slices and, once again, is stored in a protective medium until infection clearance is given.

Skin grafts are often used to assist in the healing process following severe burn injuries; heart valves are used to replace those damaged or defective through congenital abnormalities or disease; corneal and other ocular tissues are used to prevent blindness again following injury or congenital abnormality; bone, cartilage and tendons can be used to replace damaged tissue and improve quality of life (Rodrigue *et al.* 2003).

The shortage of tissue for donation is not due to a lack of potential donors, which also differentiates tissue donation from that of organ donation. Instead, it is the lack of requesting, primarily by health professionals, that has a negative impact on supply (Mack *et al.* 1995; Muraine *et al.* 2000). The publicity given to tissue donation is much less than for organs and studies point to a lack of awareness about tissue donation among the public and health professionals (Wakeford and Stepney 1989; Collins 2005; Sander and Miller 2005). Therefore lack of awareness, combined with personal attitudes and beliefs, contribute to the tissue shortage. Of all the tissue types identified in Table 6.1, it is the eye that generates the strongest attitudinal responses, as evidenced by the findings from the available literature. For this reason, although tissue in general is the focus of this chapter, attitudes to eye donation in particular will be explored. The influence of attitudes on behaviour will now be discussed.

Attitudes in general

It is generally accepted that attitudes have an effect on behaviour. In the theory of planned behaviour (Ajzen 1985, 2005) attitudes are associated with the intention to do something as well as influencing actual behaviour. Attitudinal components include cognition, affect and behaviour, which together with situational, societal and experiential factors mediate human responses to, in this case, tissue donation. So what a person believes about, how they feel about and how a person actually responds to the focus of the attitude all interact to greater or lesser degrees to influence the behavioural outcome. The affective component of attitude is bipolar with strength of feeling measured generally along a continuum ranging from strong negative to strong positive, with different aspects of donation triggering variations in attitudinal strength.

When transplantation was in its infancy, the need to understand attitudes to donation and transplantation and why people choose to donate organs or tissue generated a plethora of research. Once it became clear that, in general, attitudes to donation and transplantation were positive, the focus of attention turned to health professionals because they were, and still are, vital players in the donation process.

From the literature, it is evident that a number of factors including professional experiences, peer influence and attitudes were affecting health professionals' behavioural responses to organ and tissue donation and the donation process (Wrobbel 1989). The shortfall in supply of organs and tissue for donation persisted and in 1994 concerns were raised in the UK about the apparent reluctance of health professionals to raise the subject of donation, since this appeared to be a key contributory factor (New *et al.* 1994).

Most of the research and attention has been directed towards understanding more fully and finding solutions to the shortage of available organs for transplantation and, as a consequence, it has become apparent that health professionals differentiate between organ and tissue donation. Although health professionals have been found to hold positive attitudes to organ donation, there are aspects of the organ donation process that evoke elements of negativity, for example brain death. For tissue donation, the process is much simpler, since for most donors brain death is not a state to be determined, and other aspects generate negativity. These include the mental images arising from thoughts of eyes being retrieved and misconceptions that exist which can adversely affect health professionals' willingness to engage in the tissue donation process. The attitudes and beliefs about tissue donation and their influence on behaviour will now be discussed in more detail.

Attitudes to tissue donation

In a major survey of deaths in intensive care units in the UK, Gore *et al.* (1992) found evidence of discrepancies in donor recognition and revealed that less than 4 per cent of potential corneal donors were identified. In another survey, it was found that this is not a phenomenon unique to intensive care units; in acute care settings, deceased patients were rarely assessed for tissue donor potential (Kent 2002). In Spain, a country that has one of the highest organ donation rates in the western world, Pont *et al.* (2003) discovered that, although 25 per cent of deaths could generate potential tissue donations, less than a third of these actually result in a donation. Further evidence of problems associated with cadaveric tissue donation emerged in a UK emergency department where there was just one eye donor from 106 deaths in a 12-month period (Long *et al.* 2000).

It is recognized that tissue donation receives less attention in the media than organ donation, and this may be contributing to the general low awareness of the potential for tissue to be donated after death. Another factor is health professionals' insufficient knowledge of the processes involved and the advantages of tissue donation. Siminoff *et al.* (1995) found that most medical staff were aware of organ donor criteria, while few knew the criteria for tissues and corneas. The same has also been found in studies of nurses (Sque *et al.* 2000; Kent 2002). It may be that tissue donation does not induce the same altruistic sentiments that motivate health professionals to get involved in organ donation (Kent and Owens 1995).

Attitudes, therefore, do contribute to the non-identification of potential tissue donors. As with organ donation, the prospect of participating in donation discussions with bereaved family members is perceived as stressful and this favours non-discussion (Wakeford and Stepney 1989; Hibbert 1995). The non-discussion of tissue donation has two consequences: the loss of opportunity for the potential recipients and the loss of possible comfort during the grieving process for the bereaved family (Rodrigue *et al.* 2003).

In an attempt to understand the eye donor shortage, researchers at the University of Iowa (Mack *et al.* 1995) identified five major health professional barriers to donor eye procurement, which were:

1　Not thinking to ask.
2　Unfamiliarity with eligibility criteria.
3　Unfamiliarity with the enucleation procedure.
4　Feeling that someone else should make the request.
5　Reluctance to impose on a grieving family.

All of the above have attitudinal components. When other factors that have been identified, such as concerns about fears of disfigurement and other personal attitudes to donation, fears about the reactions of others to the discussion, and lack of experience or training in discussing such sensitive issues with bereaved families are added to the Iowa barriers (Kent and Owens 1995; Kent 2002), the extent of the influence that attitudes have on tissue donation-related behaviour becomes clear. Even though the health professional may hold positive attitudes to organ donation, tissue donation, and specifically corneal or eye donation, is viewed much less favourably. Even when it comes to considering the donation of their own, or their relatives' tissue, they are also fairly reticent. These various attitudinal factors will now be expanded upon.

Not thinking to ask

Raising awareness of the need for tissue for transplantation is indicated by the Iowa study (Mack *et al.* 1995). Odell *et al.* (1998) spoke about high awareness of organ donation but that of tissue donation is much lower with few realizing that for cases of sudden death tissue donation is a possibility that should be explored with relatives. More recent work still supports this view. Even when the death is foreseen, such as in palliative care settings, awareness of eye donation is poor, with relatives indicating that health professionals should be raising the subject with them (Carey and Forbes 2003).

Recognition that a person is a potential donor is the vital first step in the donation process for tissues and organs, since this directs future behaviour. The profiling and the strong altruistic influence of organ donation may adversely affect tissue donation. Tissue donation clearly does not receive the same level of publicity and support by transplant organizations, government agencies and the media. An American journalist suggested that loss of sight, for example, is not life-threatening so consequently does not evoke the same urgency or emotions in health professionals and the public as with organ donation (Brady 1990). The media have been influential in promoting organ donation, as reflected in the temporary upsurge in donations following national or local publicity campaigns, such as the one that was launched in Australia following the sudden death of David Hookes, a cricket icon (Mathew *et al.* 2005). The power of the media may also be influential in raising the level of awareness for tissue donation.

Unfamiliarity with the eligibility criteria

Although the eligibility criteria for tissue donation are far less complex than for organs, findings from a number of recent studies have concluded that health professionals' knowledge levels of the criteria remain poor (Kent 2002;

Hannah 2004; Collins 2005; Elding and Scholes 2005). For specific tissues, certain other criteria apply, such as age of donor and co-morbidities (see Table 6.1).

Since criteria vary, it is important that health professionals become familiar with the requirements of their local or national tissue donation service. Potential corneal tissue donors may be cared for in most hospital wards, or in fact anywhere that non-heartbeating deaths may occur; therefore, all health professionals need to be familiar with the eligibility criteria for tissue donation. They should possess the skills and knowledge needed to identify potential donors and, at the very least, to make tentative enquiries about post-death donation wishes (Matten *et al.* 1991; Sque *et al.* 2000; Kent 2004).

The lack of knowledge of the criteria for tissue donation may be due, in part, to the bias favouring organs in educational programmes. It certainly appeared to be contributing to the reluctance among nurses to begin to talk about donation with the relatives, as reflected in work by Sque who reported that one intensive care nurse in her study said: 'We're at the sharp end, meet me, teach us, support us, perhaps the yield will increase' (Sque 1996: 199). Educational programmes that aim to increase health professionals' awareness, confidence and knowledge of health concerning organ and tissue donation generally target intensive care units and so such views imply that the present system of educating and informing nurses and doctors about donation and transplantation issues may not be having the desired effect (Kent 2002, 2004).

Of all the barriers to tissue donation, lack of knowledge is one that can be successfully overcome. There is evidence worldwide that educational programmes can increase donation rates. At Israel's Sourasky Medical Centre for example, eye donation was significantly increased from 21.5 to 62 per cent of suitable candidates by increasing awareness of medical staff (Lowenstein *et al.* 1991). In a study at the Royal Melbourne Hospital Eye Bank (Chopra *et al.* 1993), a 'Gift of Sight' education and promotional programme, aimed at medical staff, resulted in requests for consent for donation being made to 323 families from 365 deaths (88.5 per cent), from which 110 corneas were retrieved in a five-month period.

Many studies have shown that an effective workshop or education programme for health care professionals that raises the profile of eye donation dramatically improves donation outcomes (Politoski and Boller 1994; Mack *et al.* 1995; Philpott *et al.* 2000). The efforts of those involved in Donor Action (in Australia) and the European Donor Hospital Education Programme (EDHEP), which are both concerned with facilitating the enhancement of communication skills with bereaved relatives require a wider audience. Attendance at EDHEP has been found to lead to significant improvement in some, but not all, communication skills that are essential when health professionals break bad news to relatives and request donation (Morton *et al.* 2000). This programme was designed in association with Eurotransplant, the overarching transplant organization covering Germany, Austria, the

Netherlands, Belgium, Luxembourg and Slovenia. Although the focus to date has been on health professionals working in critical care units, the content of the programme has far wider appeal since it provides health professionals with communication strategies that can be used with the families of deceased patients. It covers skills needed to inform about the death of a family member, appropriate responses to the family's pain and grief, informing them about the value of organ and tissue donations and finally requesting the donation itself. However, like Donor Action, because of their success in enhancing knowledge and confidence, demand for such programmes outstrips supply.

Unfamiliarity with the enucleation procedure

It is 100 years since the first corneal transplant took place (UK Transplant 2005) and despite the thousands that are performed each year across the world, health professionals continue to demonstrate a lack of awareness and knowledge of the procedures used to retrieve donated tissue from the cadaver. Misconceptions about the processes involved exist and have adversely influenced behaviour directly or indirectly. Tissue donations generally take place in the hospital mortuary or tissue donation centres, places that health professionals do not normally visit. Even when eye donations are made from deceased persons in the community setting, retrievals will often be done in funeral homes; it is the exception rather than the norm to perform the procedure in the deceased's home, although nothing precludes that happening. Consequently health professionals' exposure to the retrieval experience is low and this makes discussion about donation much harder (Odell et al. 1998).

It is clear that attitudes, particularly negative ones, can be strengthened by past experiences and for tissue donation the impact of experience is long-lasting (Kent 2004). Bad experiences of eye donation, be they actual or anecdotal, will increase the strength of negativity of attitudes to tissue donation and it is very difficult to change once established. To minimize this outcome, standards have been set in the UK for organ and tissue retrieval, to ensure that the donors are treated with respect. The process for retrieval of tissue is summarized in Figure 6.1. Consent is vital and so too is the coroner's permission, if the death has been referred to coronial services for autopsy.

Eye donation perhaps evokes the greatest or strongest negative emotions and these may be due to feelings of dissonance, personal identity and beliefs about an afterlife (Kent and Owens 1995). Dissonance arises from conflicting feelings about donation, when one favours the concept generally, but not specifically, such as eyes (Sque and Payne 1996). Issues relating to personal identity stimulate strong feelings since the eyes are thought to reflect personhood or characteristics of the person when one looks into them. They reveal, in the living, a lot about the person to whom they belong. In death,

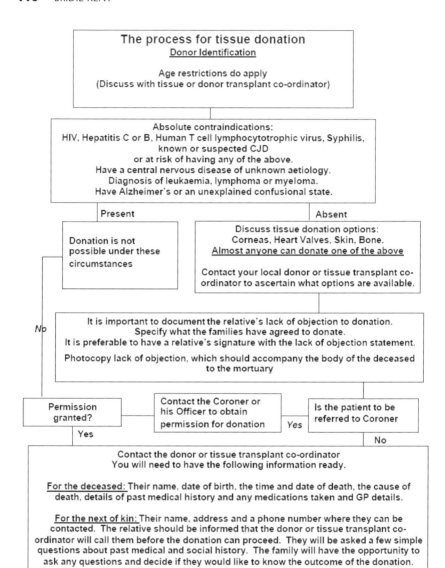

The process for tissue donation
Donor Identification

Age restrictions do apply
(Discuss with tissue or donor transplant co-ordinator)

Absolute contraindications:
HIV, Hepatitis C or B, Human T cell lymphocytotrophic virus, Syphilis,
known or suspected CJD
or at risk of having any of the above.
Have a central nervous disease of unknown aetiology.
Diagnosis of leukaemia, lymphoma or myeloma.
Have Alzheimer's or an unexplained confusional state.

Present

Donation is not
possible under these
circumstances

Absent

Discuss tissue donation options:
Corneas, Heart Valves, Skin, Bone.
Almost anyone can donate one of the above

Contact your local donor or tissue transplant co-
ordinator to ascertain what options are available.

No

It is important to document the relative's lack of objection to donation.
Specify what the families have agreed to donate.
It is preferable to have a relative's signature with the lack of objection statement.

Photocopy lack of objection, which should accompany the body of the deceased
to the mortuary

Permission
granted?

Yes

Contact the Coroner or
his Officer to obtain
permission for donation

Yes

Is the patient to be
referred to Coroner

No

Contact the donor or tissue transplant co-ordinator
You will need to have the following information ready.

For the deceased: Their name, date of birth, the time and date of death, the cause of
death, details of past medical history and any medications taken and GP details.

For the next of kin: Their name, address and a phone number where they can be
contacted. The relative should be informed that the donor or tissue transplant co-
ordinator will call them before the donation can proceed. They will be asked a few simple
questions about past medical and social history. The family will have the opportunity to
ask any questions and decide if they would like to know the outcome of the donation.

Remember the donor or tissue transplant co-ordinator is always available for advice at
any time during this process.

Figure 6.1 Tissue donation process

Source: Intensive Care Society (2004)

however, they become blank and dark and perhaps this too reinforces the state of death. Beliefs about an afterlife continue to influence behaviour and for some people the belief that eyes are needed to see into the next world remains strong (Kent and Owens 1995). Eyes have also generated sayings, many of which are a variation on 'eyes are the windows of the soul' by Thomas Phaer (c. 1510–60). For the other tissues, the emotive feelings that arise from eye donation do not appear to be nearly so influential on attitudes and behaviour.

Fear of disfigurement

Fear of disfigurement is a major barrier that also evokes strong negative attitudes among health professionals, and can be exacerbated by previous experiences. It is closely linked with the fears or misconceptions identified previously. Eyes and skin are visible and repeatedly emerge as problematic for health professionals and as tissues the public will not donate. Reasons for this phenomenon include the effect that retrieval would have on the dead body since removal of the eye or skin is perceived as being disfiguring and even disrespectful (Foy 1990). These, however, are misconceptions that can be addressed either through education or through participation in the retrieval process.

The process of tissue retrieval was described earlier and clearly every effort should be taken to ensure that the donation procedure is performed with professionalism and respect. Although it is not possible to replace the skin that has been removed and a surgical dressing does need to be applied to the donor site(s), for bone and eye donation, prostheses are inserted to ensure that disfigurement does not occur. In the case of eye donation, once the prosthesis or shell has been fitted, the eyelid remains closed by tiny hooks on the shell that grip the underneath of the lids.

The feelings of distaste or discomfort evoked when one considers the removal of tissue, particularly visible tissue such as eyes and skin, should not be dismissed as minor. Youngner (1990) suggests these are the dark sides of transplantation and they act as barriers to tissue donation. If health professionals feel strongly about this, it can prevent the discussion of donation thereby denying the relatives the opportunity to deliberate on such issues. Involvement of health professionals in the retrieval process may be one way of eradicating this belief. Concerns have also been expressed that the act of retrieval may be perceived as disrespectful to the dead body (Foy 1990) but these have to be counterbalanced in many ways by the beneficial reasons justifying the use of human tissue.

Fear of disfigurement is an important aspect of attitudes to tissue donation that affects not only health professionals but the bereaved family. They too will have questions to ask and the health professional must have the knowledge to answer these honestly and sensitively. Most of the eye banks and the tissue coordinators produce guidance information for relatives and for health professionals to assist this part of the process; they recognize that fears surrounding the retrieval are real and have a strong influence on the eventual outcome of the donation request (Chopra *et al.* 1993; Kent and Owens 1995; Doering 1996; Long *et al.* 2000).

Reluctance to impose on a grieving family

Despite the many studies that have concluded that discussions about donation, be it organ or tissue, do not increase the distress for bereaved relatives, this remains a persistent belief among health professionals. It transcends national boundaries, as evidenced by studies from the UK (Wakeford and Stepney 1989), North America (Prottas and Batten 1988) and Australia (Pearson *et al.* 2001). In a phenomenological study, Kent (2004) explored these feelings with nurses and the following quote was made by a nurse: 'The whole thing is upsetting for the family, and if they broke down on you, then you would feel really guilty, not only are you saying that they [the patient] are dying or dead but then, you aren't giving them much time to get used to the idea before the issue of donation is raised. I feel it is a lot to handle at one time' (Kent 2004: 279). Although this nurse was speaking about organ donation, with its shorter time window of opportunity in which to initiate donation discussions with relatives, other nurses identified similar recollections related to tissue donation.

The reasons for this deeply-rooted fear are complex and it appears that educational programmes, such as EDHEP have limited success in altering this belief. It may be that greater openness of donation-related discussion in society generally and specifically when a patient is admitted to acute or palliative care facilities might go some way to changing such thoughts. It is clear that health professionals find it easier to initiate donation discussions with relatives if the wishes of the deceased are known (Siminoff *et al.* 2001). The use of donor cards, driving licences and other mechanisms to record future wishes has limited use in informing health professionals of post-mortem intentions and the consensus from transplant organizations worldwide is that potential donors must discuss their intentions with their families so that their wishes are known. However, as Carey and Forbes' (2003) findings emphasized, the onus should still be on health professionals to ask about donation intentions; they should not rely on the family to raise the subject.

Fear of others' reactions

Another reason for health professionals being reluctant to raise the subject of tissue donation is fear of the reactions of other people. Relatives' responses may vary when faced with a request to consider organ or tissue donation. For example, for some, anger may be triggered and the health professional's response to this may be one of avoidance. In New Zealand, a documentary about donation and transplantation transmitted in 2005 conveyed the feelings of an intensive care specialist who stated that he was extremely reluctant to discuss donation with certain cultural groups within the population because of previous extreme reactions when donation was raised (TVNZ 2005). How widespread this type of reaction is among health professionals is not known but it does impact on donation rates since it reduces the pool of potential donors.

It is not just the reactions of relatives that are feared; so too are those of colleagues. Not knowing how others might react if, as a health professional, you indicated that a patient might be a suitable donor does act as a strong deterrent to potential involvement in the donation process. This fear might be alleviated by teamwork, especially one where all members' views are valued and respected, however, despite professional duties to act as advocates for the patients, this fear can and does inhibit future donations. As Carey and Forbes (2003) highlight, health professionals have a duty to ask.

Feeling that someone else should make the request

Hoping that someone else will do the asking for you is not uncommon. Many health professionals have experienced the mixture of feeling when faced with knowing there is a potential donor, be it organ or tissue, and that discussions with the family should now take place. Subjective aspects of caring come to the fore, and it is not uncommon for health professionals to think about themselves in that situation and ask: How would I feel? What would I want or do? The key issue to be noted here, however, is that it is not your decision. Under the law in the UK, USA and other countries where donation is operated under an opt-in policy or even as a required request, the decision can only be made by the relatives of the potential donor, or by an advanced directive if recognized by the laws of that country.

The influence of others has been described by Latané and Darley (cited by Aronson Pratkanis 1993). The focus of this research was helping behaviour within the context of emergency situations. The bystander effect was noted following the stabbing of a woman in a residential area of New York City. Despite the presence of a large number of onlookers, no assistance was given, even though the attacker was reported to have taken an hour to kill his victim. Hewstone *et al.* (1997) later referred to this phenomenon as 'bystander apathy'. Latané and Darley suggested that this phenomenon could be triggered by diffusion of responsibility and social influence. The principles of this theory may help to explain why 'caring' professionals hesitate at the thought of becoming involved in actions that would help to realize a person's post-mortem wishes.

Applying this theory to the tissue donation process, the dilemma facing the health professional is similar to that facing the bystander in the emergency situation: does he or she wait for someone else to broach the subject of tissue donation or should he or she intervene by suggesting the possibility and thus risk ridicule or embarrassment from their colleagues' unknown reactions? This may be harmful or threatening (Malecki and Hoffman 1987; Matten 1988; Wakeford and Stepney 1989). A more trusting ethos, where individual team members' opinions and actions are treated with respect could limit the bystander non-intervention effect.

The problems associated with the feeling that it is someone else's job, and discussions about donation being made by health professionals who have had limited skills and training in such matters are now widely accepted. These, together with misconceptions and misinformation have resulted in high losses of potential tissue donors. Pont *et al.* (2003) for example reported twice as many refusals for tissue donation, and losses of up to 43 per cent of potential donors. These could be directly attributed to the above issues. Studies have shown that de-coupling the discussion away from the deceased's immediate health care team has a significant effect on donation refusal rates (Williams *et al.* 2003). Therefore, the attitudinal association between the belief that someone else should make the request, and donation refusal, has been confirmed. Those health professionals, in the Iowa and other studies, were perhaps correct when they stated that they felt they were not the best people to engage in donation discussions. In response to similar data from the USA, the Federal conditions of participation (COP) for organs, tissue and eye donation were revised. These now require trained requestors to be used to make any requests for donation, and also oblige health professionals who discuss donation with potential donor families to undergo training (42 CFR Part 482 [HCFA] RIN 1998). In the UK, far greater attention is being paid to the training of health professionals and funding has been increased to allow more tissue coordinators to be appointed to assist with the donation process (UK Transplant 2005).

Protection behaviour

In essence, many of the attitudinal factors described in this chapter can be encapsulated under the term 'protection behaviours' (also see Chapter 7). Protective behaviour is common in today's world as health professionals and the general public alike try to shield themselves from some of the potentially harmful aspects of society. Protective motivation theory (Boer and Seydel 1996) has been used to explain adaptive or maladaptive processes arising from threats, vulnerability, self-efficacy and protection motivation. Another explanation for the formation of donation-related attitudes and behaviour may be avoidance, since this is behaviour that assists coping, particularly when clinicians are faced with difficult or unfamiliar circumstances (Quint 1966; McClement and Degner 1995). Avoidance behaviour is undertaken as protection against harm or hurt that might come from feelings, fears and other factors that have not been previously reconciled or faced.

There does appear to be some form of subconscious cost-benefit analysis undertaken that evaluates the risk and the benefits that might be associated with involvement in the tissue donation process. The response of health professionals to possible threats arising from the reactions of relatives, from colleagues and from their own feelings triggers a further response that will depend on the level of protection that is perceived as being required to diminish the risk of harm. It is unlikely that the health professional would feel sufficiently confident to discuss tissue donation with relatives or colleagues, if the risk of an adverse reaction is too great. Therefore, the protection element is engaged, and the subject is avoided.

The predominance of negative attitudes including beliefs, fears and misconceptions among health professionals may be explained by the need for protection. As stated earlier, experiences of donation may reinforce this protective element to behaviour. Bad experiences are more likely to evoke non-discussion behaviour, as protection from a replay of the feelings or responses that emerged from that bad experience. Good experiences, however, lessen the need for protection from these negative reactions, because they generate reactions that are congruent with the generally positive attitudes held by health professionals. These, together with training and a sufficient skill set, help the health professional to feel more confident in dealing with any emotions that may arise from the donation discussion. Conversely, negative attitudes and poor knowledge may similarly be used to justify non-discussion behaviour.

While Pilsworth (1994) argued that, for some circumstances or individuals, distancing or other defence strategies might be beneficial by facilitating coping, the effect of these actions, if used inappropriately, may be less satisfactory. If protective behaviours are employed in every circumstance when the discussion of donation intentions is appropriate, the shortfall in availability of donated tissue would worsen.

In a study of nurses' post-mortem experiences, Wolf (1990, 1994) concluded that although involvement in post-mortem care of whatever variety was emotionally draining, the health professionals (nurses in this case) still saw it as a worthwhile and necessary part of health care. The decision-making process forces us to question the key factors that underlie our choice of action. Payne *et al.* (1993) argue that we assess a potential outcome in terms of its being a 'good' decision, while at the same time assessing the degree of cognitive effort that is required; compromises may have to be made.

The attitudinal barriers identified here can be overcome. The evidence overwhelmingly points to a willingness by health professionals for greater involvement in the organ donation process, and one would hope that this also extends to tissue donation. It may be that getting others engaged, such as transplant coordinators or nominated trained requestors, rather than relying on the health professionals to initiate donation discussions, may be the way forward. However, these can only be brought in once the potential, in this case for tissue donation, has been identified. Health professionals therefore do need to be aware of the effect of their attitudes to tissue donation on subsequent behaviour, consider the need for further training especially where knowledge deficits have been identified, and become more aware of the increasing and persistent need for human tissue for transplantation. There are indications that behaviour is changing. Student doctors and nurses appear to have more strongly positive attitudes to donation than their qualified counterparts (Cantwell and Clifford 2000; Essman and Lebovitz 2005) and their knowledge of aspects of the donation process was better than, or equal to, registered nurses (Kent 1998).

Conclusion

The attitudes of health professionals to tissue donation and the supply of human tissue for transplantation are clearly closely associated. Given the growing need to ensure that eyes, heart valves, bone and skin are available for transplantation surgery, there is a need for health professionals to have a much greater awareness of this form of cadaveric donation. The public have indicated their support for organ donation and those who are aware that eyes and other forms of tissue can be donated after death show similar levels of endorsement.

The media and transplant organizations could certainly do more to educate society about tissue donation, and efforts being made to include this topic into undergraduate medical and nursing programmes appear to be successful. Therefore it is possible that future health professionals will not hold the beliefs and fears that become apparent when their qualified colleagues' attitudes are studied. However, all that takes time. For the present and immediate future, today's health professionals need to rise to the challenge. By raising awareness of the influence of attitudes on donation rates, by addressing the issues identified in this chapter and through increasing publicity, it should be possible to increase the supply of donated tissue. An active policy for corneal donation in an emergency department saw a dramatic increase in donation rates from 1 per cent to 35 per cent.

De-coupling also appears to be effective but Williams *et al.* (2003) did warn of the danger of alienating the 'non-trained' health professionals as a result of this process. Knowing the patient's wishes may make a difference to the relatives and this knowledge can also alleviate some of the concerns of health professionals (Siminoff and Lawrence 2002; Rodrigue *et al.* 2006). However, a study by Sque *et al.* (2006) found that at times families do go against their decedent's wishes.

Ultimately, the decision to donate remains, in many parts of the world, a matter of personal choice and one that is made for many different reasons. The decision of the health professional to ask about post-mortem wishes has far-reaching implications for potential recipients of the tissue, and may have benefits for family and friends of the deceased. Perkins *et al.* (2005: 711) stated emphatically that 'excellent end of life care extends beyond death', therefore health professionals have a duty to consider the wishes of the patient and family, and to help those relatives to make the appropriate end of life decision that is right for them.

References

42 CFR Part 482 [HCFA] RIN (1998) 0938-A195 Medicare and Medicaid programmes; hospital conditions of participation; identification of potential organ, tissue and eye donors and transplant hospitals' provision of transplant-related data: HCFA. Final Rule, *Federal Register*, 63: 33856–7.

Ajzen, I. (1985) From intentions to actions: a theory of planned behaviour, in J. Kuhl and J. Beckmann (eds) *Action Control: from Cognition to Behaviour*. New York: Springer-Verlag.

Ajzen, I. (2005) *Attitudes, Personality, and Behavior*, 2nd edn. Maidenhead: Open University Press.

Aronson, E. and Pratkanis, A.R. (eds) (1993) *Social Psychology*. Aldershot: Edward Elgar.

Boer, H. and Seydel, E. (1996) Protective motivation theory, in M. Conner and P. Norman (eds) *Predictive Health Behaviour: Research and Practice with Social Cognition Models*. Buckingham: Open University Press.

Brady, W. (1990) Role of the media in organ donation, *Transplantation Proceedings*, 22(3): 1047–9.

Cantwell, M. and Clifford, C. (2000) English nursing and medical students' attitudes toward organ donation, *Journal of Advanced Nursing*, 32: 961–8.

Carey, I. and Forbes, K. (2003) The experience of donor families in the hospice, *Palliative Medicine*, 17: 241–7.

Chopra, G.K., De Vincentis, F., Kaufman, D. and Collie, D. (1993) Effective corneal retrieval in a general hospital: The Royal Melbourne Hospital Eye Bank, *Australian and New Zealand Journal of Ophthalmology*, 21: 251–5.

Collins, T. J. (2005) Organ and tissue donation: a survey of nurse's knowledge and educational needs in an adult ITU, *Intensive & Critical Care Nursing*, 21(4): 226–33.

Cunningham, M., Majzoub, R., Brouha, P., Laurentin-Perez, L.A., Naidu, D.K., Maldonado, C., Banis, J.C., Frank, J.M. and Barker, J.H. (2004) Risk acceptance in composite tissue allotransplantation reconstructive procedures, *European Journal of Trauma*, 30: 12–16.

Devauchelle, B., Badet, L., Lengele, B., Morelon, E., Testelin, S., Michallet, M., D'Hauthuille, C. and Dubernard, J. (2006) First human face allograft: early report, *The Lancet*, 368: 203–9.

Doering, J.J. (1996) Families experiences in consenting to eye donation of a recently deceased relative, *Heart and Lung*, 25(1): 72–8.

Elding, C. and Scholes, J. (2005) Organ and tissue donation: a trustwide perspective or critical care concern? *Nursing in Critical Care*, 10(3): 129–35.

Essman, C.C. and Lebovitz, D.J. (2005) Donation education for medical students: enhancing the link between physicians and procurement professionals, *Progress in Transplantation*, 15(2): 124–8.

Foy, J.M. (1990) Duty to respect the dead body: a nursing perspective, *Transplantation Proceedings*, 22(3): 1023–4.

Gore, S.M., Cable, D.J. and Holland, A.J. (1992) Organ donation from intensive care units in England and Wales: a two year confidential audit of deaths in intensive care, *British Medical Journal*, 304: 349–55.

Hannah, S. (2004) Increasing awareness of tissue donation: in the non-heart beating donor, *Intensive & Critical Care Nursing*, 20(5): 292–8.

Hewstone, M., Manstead, A. and Stroebe, W. (1997) *The Blackwell Reader in Social Psychology*. Oxford: Blackwell.

Hibbert, M. (1995) Stressors experienced by nurses while caring for organ donors and their families, *Heart and Lung*, 24(5): 399–407.

Intensive Care Society (2004) *Guidelines for Organ and Tissue Donation*, www. ics.ac.uk/downloads/Standards/Master%20ICS%20Guidelines%20all%20 sections%20(Nov04).pdf (accessed 10 May 2006).

Kann, B.R., Furnas, D.W. and Hewitt, C.W. (2000) Past, present and future research in the field of composite tissue allotransplantation, *Microsurgery*, 20(8): 393–9.

Kent, B. (1998) *Organ and tissue donation: factors influencing nurses' willingness to discuss post mortem donation wishes*. Ph.D. thesis, University of Wales, Bangor, Wales.

Kent, B. (2002) Psychosocial factors influencing nurses' involvement with organ and tissue donation, *International Journal of Nursing Studies*, 39: 429–40.

Kent, B. (2004) Protection behaviour: a phenomenon affecting organ and tissue donation in the 21st century? *International Journal of Nursing Studies*, 41(3): 273–84.

Kent, B. and Owens, R. G. (1995) Conflicting attitudes to corneal and organ donation: a study of nurses' attitudes to organ donation, *International Journal of Nursing Studies*, 32(5): 484–92.

Long, J., Walsh, D., Ritchie, D.A.W. and Russell, F. (2000) Corneal donation in the accident and emergency department: observational study, *British Medical Journal*, 321: 1263–4.

Lowenstein, A., Rahmiel, R., Carssano, D. and Moshe, L. (1991) Obtaining consent for eye donation, *Israel Journal of Medical Science*, 27: 79–81.

Mack, R., Mason, P. and Mathers, W. (1995) Obstacles to donor eye procurement and their solutions at the University of Iowa, *Cornea*, 14(3): 249–52.

Malecki, M.R. and Hoffman, M.C. (1987) Getting to yes: how nurses' attitudes affect their success in obtaining consent for organ and tissue donation, *Dialysis and Transplantation*, 16: 276–8.

Mathew, T., Faull, R. and Snelling, P. (2005) The shortage of kidneys for transplantation in Australia, *Medical Journal of Australia*, 182(5): 204–5.

Matten, M.R. (1988) *Nurses' knowledge, attitudes and beliefs about organ and tissue donation and transplantation*. Ph.D. thesis, Southern Illinois University, USA.

Matten, M.R., Sliepcevich, E.M., Sarvela, P.D., Lacey, E.P., Woehike, P.L., Richardson, C.E. and Wright, W.R. (1991) Nurses' knowledge, attitudes and beliefs regarding organ and tissue donation and transplantation, *Public Health Reports*, 106(2): 155–66.

McClement, S.E. and Degner, L.F. (1995) Expert nursing behaviours in care of the dying adult in the intensive care unit, *Heart and Lung*, 24(5): 408–19.

Metropolitan Health and Aged Services Division (2004) *Hospital Circulars 2004: Provision of Patient Information to the Lions Corneal Donation Service*. Melbourne: Victorian State Government Department of Human Services.

Morton, J., Blok, G., Reid, C., van Dalen, J. and Morley, M. (2000) The European Donor Hospital Education Programme (EDHEP): enhancing communication skills with bereaved relatives, *Anaesthesia and Intensive Care*, 28(2): 184–90.

Muraine, M., Menguy, E., Martin, J., Sabatier, P., Watt, L. and Brasseur, G. (2000) The interview with the donor's family before postmortem cornea procurement, *Cornea*, 19(1): 12–16.

New, B., Solomon, M., Solomon, M., Dingwall, R. and McHale, J. (1994) *A Question of Give and Take: Improving the Supply of Donor Organs for Transplantation*. London: King's Fund Institute.

Odell, J., Boyce, S. and Siddall, S. (1998) Tissue viability supplement: tissue donation – the benefit of a positive approach, *Nursing Standard*, 13(3): 66–71.

Payne, J.W., Bettman, J.R. and Johnson, E.J. (1993) Deciding how to decide: an effort-accuracy framework, in J.W. Payne, J.R. Bettman and E.J. Johnson (eds) *The Adaptive Decision Maker*. Cambridge, MA: Cambridge University Press.

Pearson, A., Robertson-Malt, S., Walsh, K. and FitzGerald, M. (2001) Intensive care nurses' experiences of caring for brain dead organ donor patients, *Journal of Clinical Nursing*, 10(1): 132–9.

Perkins, H.S., Shepherd, K.J., Cortez, J.D. and Hazuda, H.P. (2005) Exploring chronically ill seniors' attitudes about discussing death and postmortem medical procedures, *Journal of the American Geriatrics Society*, 53(5): 895–900.

Philpott, M., Bain, M. and Coster, D.J. (2000) Procurement of all the cornea donors needed: how is it achieved? *Transplantation Proceedings*, 32: 69–71.

Pilsworth, T. (1994) Dying is a normal process whether or not resulting from disease, *Journal of Cancer Care*, 3(1): 2–11.

Politoski, G. and Boller, J. (1994) Making the critical difference: an innovative approach to educating nurses about organ and tissue donation, *Critical Care Nursing Clinics of North America*, 6(3): 581–5.

Pont, T., Gracia, R.M., Valdes, C., Nieto, C., Rodellar, L., Arancibia, I. and Deulofeu Vilarnau, R. (2003) Theoretic rates of potential tissue donation in a university hospital, *Transplantation Proceedings*, 35(5): 1640–1.

Prottas, J. and Batten, H.L. (1988) Health professionals and hospital administrators in organ procurement: attitudes, reservations and their resolutions, *American Journal of Public Health*, 78(6): 642–5.

Quint, J. (1966) Awareness of death and the nurse's composure, *Nursing Research*, 15(1): 49–55.

Rodrigue, J.R., Scott, M.P. and Oppenheim, A.R. (2003) The tissue donation experience: a comparison of donor and nondonor families, *Progress in Transplantation*, 13(4): 258–64.

Rodrigue, J.R., Cornell, D.L. and Howard, R.J. (2006) Organ donation decision: comparison of donor and nondonor families, *American Journal of Transplantation*, 6(1): 190–8.

Sander, S.L. and Miller, B.K. (2005) Public knowledge and attitudes regarding organ and tissue donation: an analysis of the northwest Ohio community, *Patient Education & Counseling*, 58(2): 154–63.

Siminoff, L.A. and Lawrence, R. (2002) Knowing patients' preferences about organ donation: does it make a difference? *Journal of Trauma Injury, Infection and Critical Care*, 53: 754–60.

Siminoff, L.A., Arnold, R.M. and Caplan, A.L. (1995) Health care professionals' attitudes towards donation: effect on practice and procurement, *The Journal of Trauma*, 39(3): 553–9.

Siminoff, L.A., Gordon, N., Hewlett, J. and Arnold, R. (2001) Factors influencing families' consent for donation of solid organs for transplantation, *Journal of the American Medical Association*, 286(1): 71–7.

Sque, M. (1996) *The experiences of donor relatives, and nurses' attitudes, knowledge and behaviour regarding cadaveric donotransplantation.* Ph.D. thesis, University of Southampton, Southampton: UK.

Sque, M. and Payne, S. (1996) Dissonant loss: the experiences of donor relatives, *Social Science & Medicine*, 43(9): 1359–70.

Sque, M., Payne, S. and Vlachonikolis, L. (2000) Cadaveric donotransplantation:

Nurses' attitudes, knowledge and behaviour, *Social Science & Medicine*, 50: 541–52.

Sque, M., Long, T., Payne, S. and Allardyce, D. (2006) *Exploring the End of Life Decision-making and Hospital Experiences of Families Who Did Not Donate Organs for Transplant Operations. Final Research Report for UK Transplant*. University of Southampton, Southampton: UK.

TVNZ (2005) *DNZ: The Waiting List*, 20 June 2005. www.bsa.govt.nz/decisions/ 2005/2005–101.htm (accessed 10 May 2006).

UK Transplant (2005) *UK Transplant Business Plan 2005–2006*. Bristol: UK Transplant.

Wakeford, R.E. and Stepney, R. (1989) Obstacles to organ donation, *British Journal of Surgery*, 76(5): 435–9.

Williams, M.A., Lipsett, P.A., Rushton, C.H., Grochowski, E.C., Berkowitz, I., Mann, S.L., Shatzer, J.H., Short, M.P. and Genel, M. (2003) The physician's role in discussing organ donation with families, *Critical Care Medicine*, 31(5): 1568–73.

Wolf, Z.R. (1990) Nurses' experiences giving post mortem care to patients who have donated organs: a phenomenological study, *Transplantation Proceedings*, 22(3): 1019–20.

Wolf, Z.R. (1994) Nurses' responses to organ procurement from non-beating cadaver donors, *AORN*, 60(6): 968–81.

Wrobbel, P. A. (1989) Anatomical gift donation, *Orthopaedic Nursing*, 8(2): 26–9.

Youngner, S. J. (1990) Organ Retrieval: can we ignore the dark side? *Transplantation Proceedings*, 22(3): 1014–15.

7 Facilitating the donation discussion beyond intensive care: lessons from specialist palliative care

Joanne Wells, Delyth Hughes and Parul Mistry

Introduction

With an increasing gap between the demand for donated organs and tissues for transplantation and the available supply, there is a need to facilitate donation from clinical environments other than intensive care. In this chapter we draw mainly on UK data to highlight the potential for donation from alternative settings such as accident and emergency departments, general wards, the primary care setting and palliative care units. Initially we will discuss the possibilities and problems associated with non-heartbeating donation.[1] We will then focus on non-heartbeating donation from the palliative care setting, examining the current literature, particularly studies by two of the authors (Wells and Hughes). Finally we will highlight the issues influencing donation from non-heartbeating donors who die outside the intensive care unit, and pinpoint the differences that exist between donation from this setting and the palliative care environment.

Beyond intensive care: possibilities and problems

Possibilities

Prior to establishment of brain death criteria (Ad Hoc Harvard Committee 1968) non-heartbeating donors were the only source of organs and tissues. With the introduction of the legal definition of brain death, brain dead patients became a more preferred source of organs. Practical concerns regarding warm ischaemia, the amount of time the organ spends at room temperature without any oxygen supply and organ preservation were principle drawbacks, making non-heartbeating donation impractical (Kimber *et al.* 2001). However, advances in medical technology and organ and tissue preservation have now made donation from non-heartbeating donors a more viable option. The declining incidence of brain death, in part due to the drop in catastrophic brain injury, and its improved neuro-critical care management, also means that non-heartbeating donation offers great potential for expansion of the donor pool.

While strict donor criteria confine most solid organ donation to heart-beating patients maintained on ventilators in intensive care units, individuals who die in other clinical areas can potentially donate a variety of tissues, and occasionally solid organs, such as kidneys, for transplantation. Although the majority of kidneys transplanted are from heartbeating or live donors, successful transplants have also been performed using kidneys from non-heartbeating donors. Thus, with recent figures showing over 5000 patients in the UK and 67,003 people in the USA on the active kidney transplant waiting list, there has been renewed interest in the retrieval of kidneys from patients who have already suffered cardio-respiratory arrest. To reduce the risk of damage to the kidney, retrieval needs to take place quickly and in an operating theatre (Lewis and Valerius 1999; Kimber *et al.* 2001). Thus, although the donation of kidneys is theoretically possible from areas other than intensive care, in practice it is usually restricted to either the intensive care setting or the accident and emergency environment. However, if patient, family and health professionals were all properly prepared, perhaps it might be possible to transfer suitable patients from the general ward to the operating theatre immediately following death.

Although as Kent (Chapter 6) pointed out, tissue donation does not enjoy the same high public profile as organ donation (Odell *et al.* 1998) it nevertheless holds many significant benefits for recipients. Tissue donation is also subject to fewer contra-indications and restrictions than are associated with solid organ donation, retrieval times are less urgent, varying from between up to 24 hours after death for corneas, to 48 hours for heart valves. According to UK Transplant (2004), many patients who die in clinical environments outside intensive care have the potential to be non-heartbeating corneal donors, while those with non-malignancies may be able to donate a variety of tissues such as heart valves, bone and skin, as well as corneas.

Problems

Despite the fact that many patients in a variety of clinical settings could be non-heartbeating donors, statistics suggest that only limited donation takes place in areas other than the intensive care settings (Gore *et al.* 1992; Sque *et al.* 2000; Wells and Sque 2002). Plausible reasons for this seemingly low commitment to donation include the controversies surrounding the definition of death for a non-heartbeating donor. This is particularly an issue when considering organ donation from patients who have died through a sudden event. The struggle to ensure that the organs removed are viable for transplantation, and that the patient was dead at the time the organs were removed, remain major areas of concern. The two major issues that bioethicists have grappled with, in non-heartbeating donor protocol, include timing of death and definition of irreversibility. There are no definitive studies or protocols which provide guidance regarding the optimal waiting time after the heart stops beating. Variable waiting times from 2 minutes to 10 minutes after cessation of the heartbeat have been proposed and practised by different institutions (Robinson 1912; Enselberg 1952; Rodstein and Bornstein 1970; Quick and Bastani 1994; Institute of Medicine 1997).

Another hotly debated topic revolves around the *irreversible* loss of cardiac function, proposed in the definition of death for non-heartbeating donors (Institute of Medicine 1997; Youngner *et al.* 1999; Doig and Rocker 2003). It raises questions of '*irreversible*' as declared by whom, when and under what circumstances. There are no medical or legal texts that specify the real time of death.

Another reason for the seemingly low commitment is health care professionals' failure to either identify potential donors or to introduce opportunities that might allow the donation process to take place (Gore *et al.* 1992; Sque *et al.* 2000). These reasons are given credence by the results of studies investigating the knowledge and attitudes towards donotransplantation[2] of health care professionals in different clinical settings. Sque *et al.* (2000), for example, compared the knowledge, attitudes and behaviour of UK nurses, regarding donotransplantation, working in a variety of clinical settings. Postal questionnaires were sent to 2465 nurses working on general medical and surgical wards, accident and emergency departments, operating theatres, intensive care units and renal dialysis and transplant units. A 54 per cent response rate (n = 1333) was achieved. Results showed that renal dialysis and transplant nurses, followed by intensive care nurses, held the most positive views about the donotransplantation process. They also placed more importance on donation than nurses from other clinical settings and did not perceive that discussion about donation would increase families' distress. Conversely, nurses working in the operating theatre and on general wards were the least positive about donation, were more concerned about its interventionist and mutilating aspects, and believed that discussion about the subject with relatives would increase their distress.

Sque *et al.* concluded that while intensive care and renal dialysis and transplant nurses were both knowledgeable and supportive of the donation process, there was evidence of complacency regarding donation among accident and emergency nurses and negative attitudes among those working on general wards. This led the authors to propose that nurses who are involved with the donotransplantation process may have a more empathic response, and thus be more positive about donation. Conversely, those who are not knowledgeable, and have no experience of the process, are likely to be more negative, possibly because they are not expected to consider facilitation of the donation process as part of their role. The results of this study are supported by those of Bridgare and Oermann (1991) and Garde and Corbett (1994) who found that nurses who had experience of donation, either personally or professionally, held more positive attitudes than those who had no experience. Furthermore, Wells and Sque (2002) found that palliative care professionals who had little or no experience of the donation process were concerned that donation discussion would increase the distress of relatives.

Nurses' attitudes to and knowledge about donation, and their clinical speciality, may not be the only factors to influence the donation process. What is not known is how the process is affected by issues such as the patient's cause of death and/or the clinical environment where they die. When a patient dies in an intensive care unit the death is often sudden and unexpected and, unless the patient has made their wishes with regard to donation explicit prior to admission, they are unlikely to be able to be involved in the decision-making process. Outside the intensive care environment patients may die after a long illness, with death an anticipated outcome, enabling potential involvement in discussions about whether or not they wish to be a donor. Does the fact that death is expected alter the decisions made by patients and families with regard to donation, or the bereavement processes of families? Possible answers to these questions may be found by considering research from the palliative care environment. Such consideration may also be useful in enhancing understanding of the low commitment to donation by health professionals in both the palliative care and other clinical areas.

The palliative care experience

Palliative care can be defined as 'the active holistic care of patients with advanced progressive disease' (WHO 2002: 83) and together with the management of physical symptoms and the provision of psychosocial and spiritual support, ensures patients have adequate information to make informed choices. These have always been considered fundamental principles of palliative care (National Council for Hospice and Palliative Care Services 1995; National Institute for Clinical Excellence 2004). However, despite priding themselves on their ability to communicate with patients, involving them in their care, and having the skills and expertise to explore sensitive issues (Feuer 1998; Kennedy 2003; Clover *et al.* 2004; Mok and Chiu 2004), research suggests that palliative care professionals do not give any greater consideration to the facilitation of donation than colleagues working in other clinical areas (Spivey 1998; Wells and Sque 2002). Spivey (1998) demonstrated this point through the results of a questionnaire sent to 55 per cent (n = 83) of the palliative care units in England. It was found that of the 33 units who believed that donation was appropriate only 2 reported that they routinely discussed donation with patients and families.

Although patients who die of non-curable illnesses in specialist palliative care units and hospices cannot be multi-organ donors, they can potentially, like other groups of patients outside intensive care, donate a variety of tissues and, rarely, their kidneys. In practice, corneas are the most common tissue to be donated. This is because the majority of palliative care patients have a cancer diagnosis and, unlike most other organs and tissues, a cancer diagnosis does not preclude corneal donation. Also, the process is relatively simple and can take place within the clinical area, at a mortuary or an undertaker (Wells and Sque 2002).

Research from the palliative care setting

Currently, although a wealth of literature exists in relation to donation from within the intensive care setting, very little stems from any other clinical setting. Sque *et al.* (2000) and Sque and Wells (2004) believe that this paucity reflects the fact that intensive care is still generally considered to be the only place where discussion about organ and tissue donation takes place. However, where research outside intensive care does exist it appears to stem mainly from the palliative care setting. This may be because palliative care professionals, espousing the ethos of care described above, feel uncomfortable about, and thus wish to investigate, anything they perceive to be undermining patients' right to autonomous informed choice.

In the earliest published work on organ donation in the hospice setting, Peters and Sutcliffe (1992) retrospectively reviewed patients' records to present an account of 12 non-heartbeating kidney donors who died in St Christopher's Hospice, London, between January 1990 and October 1991. The positive effects for patients and families were discussed and the issues for staff explored. Being the first of its kind, this study was valuable in stimulating thought and discussion among health care professionals about the possibility of donation. However, since it was published the criteria for kidney donation have changed and, for the reasons described earlier in this chapter, kidney donation from patients who die in hospices and palliative care units rarely happens.

A more recent study by Carey and Forbes (2003) explored the experiences, attitudes and feelings of relatives who consented to the donation of the corneas of loved ones who had died of cancer within a palliative care setting.

Ten donor relatives were interviewed between 4 to 12 months after their family member's death. The findings showed that, generally, the experience was considered positively by the donor families. It also showed that the majority of participants believed, due to cancer or old age, that their family member was ineligible for donation. Thus, had the subject not been raised with them by a palliative care professional, they would never have considered donation to be an option. The family members also indicated that donation decisions were easier if patient's wishes were known prior to death. This was a small study with data from two palliative care units. However, it supported previous research carried out within the critical care environment, high-lighting both the gatekeeping role of health care professionals in facilitating donation, and the potential positive effects for bereaved families (Sque and Payne 1994).

Carey and Forbes' (2003) study confirmed and expanded on many of the findings of the study by Wells and Sque (2002) who investigated why the commitment to tissue donation in specialist palliative care units is low. Eight nurses and two doctors, employed within two specialist palliative care units, participated in semi-structured interviews to explore their views, feelings and experiences of tissue donation. The findings suggested that while in theory palliative care professionals thought it appropriate to approach patients re-garding donation, thus supporting Spivey's (1998) study, they feared that raising the subject could cause distress and psychological harm. This was because talking about donation required the professional to broach the sub-ject of the patient's death, an issue which even the palliative care staff felt uncomfortable about. Furthermore, the authors found these issues and con-cerns were interwoven with the levels of knowledge and confidence the participants had about donation, which consequently affected their profes-sional role in regard to donation. Wells and Sque concluded that the unique ability of palliative care patients to make their own decisions about donation had many implications and concerns for the health professionals who cared for them. They described this as the theory of 'living choice' which they defined as '*The ability of terminally ill patients within the palliative care en-vironment to make choices about donation that have an impact on the knowledge and role of health professionals*' (p. 24).

Although a small, qualitative study, Wells and Sque's work highlighted many issues for discussion and emphasized some of the differences between intensive care and palliative care settings. Perhaps the most significant of these was the ability of patients within the latter environment to be involved in the decision-making process about donation and the implications that this appeared to have on the professional role in facilitating donation.

Of the three studies published so far, none have taken into account the views of, arguably, the most important stakeholder in the donation process: the patient. To address this gap Hughes (2005), in a small qualitative study, explored the knowledge and attitudes of palliative care patients with regard to organ and tissue donation. The study highlighted the impact, on them, of donation discussion and thus the potential implications for practice. Eight patients attending a specialist palliative care day centre participated in face-to-face interviews and discussed subjects such as their general attitudes towards organ and tissue donotransplantation, their knowledge of donation criteria, how they felt when the subject of donation was raised with them (and perceived other patients might feel), and their views on if, when, how and by whom information about their potential donation choices should be given to them.

Five categories: 'talking', 'not knowing', 'considering', 'coping' and 'finding the right way' were elicited from the data and intertwined to support a tentative new theory, 'evocative talk'. This captured the essence of the data and was defined as: *'The nature of the organ/tissue donation discussion which, when raised with palliative care patients, assumes a greater significance than it might for other groups of patients or the general public and has the potential, therefore, to be hope hindering, hope enhancing or both'* (p. 40).

The theory, as the definition suggests, highlighted that while the donation discussion may, by counteracting some of the negative psychosocial factors associated with terminal disease, be experienced very positively by patients, and have the potential to increase the donor pool, it may, by challenging the coping mechanisms used to manage the threat of imminent death, also cause distress. The author concluded that while palliative care professionals should not exclude a donation discussion from the list of important end of life issues that need addressing with patients, they need also to develop strategies that will enable accurate judgements to be made regarding the appropriateness of this for individual patients.

As stated previously, evidence suggests that depending on their knowledge and commitment to the donation process, nurses and doctors control access to potential donors and thus are 'gatekeepers' to the process (Sque and Payne 1994; Kent 2002; Wells and Sque 2002). With this in mind, Wells (2004), building on her earlier study (Wells and Sque 2002), is expanding the variety of informants to elicit the views of not only palliative care doctors and nurses, but also chaplaincy teams, social workers, palliative care patients, bereaved families, recipients of corneas and members of donotransplant teams. Preliminary analysis of 11 interviews suggests that gatekeeping by health professionals may, in part, derive from a desire to *'protect from harm all those affected by the donation process'* (Wells 2004: 44), a phenomenon the author describes as 'shielding behaviour'.

This desire is multi-faceted and, although it conflicts with the participants' knowledge of the potential benefits of donation, is nevertheless repeatedly referred to. It includes firstly the desire to protect patients and relatives from conversations that may broach the subject of the patient's death, secondly, believing that the maintenance of a physically intact body may be necessary for the protection of the patient's physical 'being' and identity, thirdly, wishing to protect the traditional palliative care ideal of a 'good, natural death' from the process of donotransplantation, which is steeped in medical technology, and, finally, protecting the individual practitioner from the requirement to promote a subject that may conflict with their personal values and beliefs. Wells' (2004) findings appear to be consistent with those of Kent (2004) who, in a study in the acute setting of nurses' attitudes and behaviours towards donation discussion, found that nurses desired to protect not only patients but also relatives, colleagues and themselves from any distress that might be engendered from such a discussion.

Discussion

The psychosocial impact of terminal disease has been widely commented upon. Charmaz (1980) suggests that the debilitating symptoms of advancing disease displace the terminally ill from social roles and functions, resulting in loss of self-identity. Similarly Copp (1999) believes that dying people experience grief as they face progressive loss of control, while Madioni et al. (1997) suggest that deterioration in physical function and independence may engender feelings of shame and humiliation.

The results of Hughes' (2005) study suggest that the provision of information about donor eligibility to terminally ill patients may have positive benefits. Feasibly, not only might it have the potential to increase the availability of tissues (and occasional kidneys) for transplantation but, for dying patients, it may facilitate autonomy and, by providing a new purpose in life, an attainable goal, and the satisfaction of knowing that (despite terminal disease) they can still contribute to society, counteract some of the negative psychosocial factors described above, thus increasing psychological well-being. Furthermore, Carey's and Forbes' (2003) findings suggest that facilitating the wish of a loved one to be a donor may be a positive experience for relatives and could have possible long-term positive effects on their bereavement.

The results of these two studies also suggest that palliative care patients and their families are likely to presume that a diagnosis of cancer precludes the patient from being eligible as a donor. Similar misconceptions about donor criteria (such as exclusion due to age and other medical conditions) have been found in research with the general public (Basu et al. 1989; Gallup 1993). It seems possible, therefore, that this lack of knowledge could extend to other potential donors, such as those with life-limiting conditions other than cancer and/or those with chronic diseases, in environments such as general wards or primary care. Furthermore, knowledge of eligibility to donate may bring patients in these groups the same kind of psychological benefits as those dying of cancer.

In view of the above it seems reasonable to expect that if health care professionals, both in palliative care and in other clinical specialities, are to facilitate autonomy for their patients, and grant them the potential benefits as described above, as well as increasing the numbers of tissues for donation, they need to provide patients with information regarding their options to be a donor. Indeed, it could perhaps even be argued that not to do so breaches their professional role. However, while this argument is compelling, it should not be forgotten that the terminally ill participants in Hughes' (2005) study advocated against a blanket policy of uniformly discussing donation with every patient (at the same time and in the same way); a caution that was endorsed by palliative care professionals in the studies by Sque and Wells (2004) and Wells (2004), thus giving some justification to the intuitive concerns of palliative care professionals that they might cause psychological harm. It is important, therefore, instead of advocating a blanket policy of discussion with all patients, to consider why certain patients might be distressed and to take a more individualistic approach.

The premise that, in western society, death is considered taboo has recently been the subject of some debate and it has been argued that with changing attitudes towards death, individuals are becoming more able to talk openly and freely about the subject (Walters 1993; Rinopoche 1995; O'Gorman 1998). Indeed, one of the key figures in forging this change in attitude was the hospice movement pioneer, Dame Cicely Saunders, who in the 1960s set about improving the care provided to the terminally ill by addressing the difficulties encountered by patients, families and health professionals and encouraged working in partnership with patients to facilitate autonomy and ensure their wishes were met. However, the ability to talk openly about death may depend on many factors and, for the terminally ill participants in Hughes' study, it appeared that talking about a death-related subject such as donation, by forcing them to focus on the future, had the capacity to interfere with the coping strategies (such as denial) they used to deal psychologically with the prospect of an imminent death. Hughes (2005) suggests, therefore, that whether taboo or not, death may still be a frightening prospect for many individuals and thus the degree to which they are able to engage comfortably in discussion about it may depend on the extent to which they are able to depersonalize and distance themselves from death's reality. The results of Hughes' study suggested that this is likely to be difficult for some terminally ill patients for whom the future is uncertain and who want, therefore, as Lawton (2000) suggests, to ignore this temporal framework, preferring instead to focus on past or present concerns. However, arguably this may not be the case for patients with non life-threatening and/or chronic illnesses who, like healthy individuals, may still be able to cling to the 'myth of immortality' (Nekolaichuk and Bruera 1998), wherein time is perceived as endless, hope is firmly linked with the future and thus death can be considered a distant and vague concept.

Even if it is felt that a particular patient may not be distressed talking about donation, the extent to which patients and their families wish to be involved in decision-making regarding their care varies enormously (Degner and Sloane 1992; Thompson *et al.* 1993; Bruera *et al.* 2001). Thus, if health care professionals are to accept that giving information to patients about donation is part of their professional role it seems they will be required to make accurate and balanced decisions as to when and with whom donation discussion should happen, or, if not appropriate, consider by which alternative methods information might be given. This decision-making process may be facilitated by considering the responses of the participants in both Hughes' (2005) and Wells' (2004) studies. Both the palliative care patients and health care professionals identified 'knowing' an individual patient to be vital in ascertaining whether or not they might be distressed by a discussion of donation. Similarly, when asked to consider who might be an appropriate person to raise the subject (if indeed it is to be raised at all), the consensus of the participants in both studies was that it should be a professional who had developed a good rapport with the patient and knew him or her well.

Within the fields of oncology and palliative care, Maguire (1999) and Ronaldson and Devery (2001) suggest that a key skill in facilitating the decision-making process is the extent to which health care professionals can both identify with the information needs of patients and are able to pick up cues that lead to the initiation of information exchange at an appropriate time and suitable level for the patient. Similarly, in relation to donation, the key appears to lie in the ability of health care professionals to build, through the development of a trusting relationship, an in-depth knowledge of individual patients that will allow them accurately to predict their likely reaction to the donation discussion. Copp (1999) suggests that nurses looking after terminally ill patients often form close emotional bonds. Similarly, Murray *et al.* (2004) believe that hospice nurses understand that patients possess important self-knowledge. Thus, understanding what represents the best choices for them is pivotal in providing relevant, accurate information. It is quite likely that nurses working in other settings, such as the community, general wards and nursing homes may also form such bonds with their patients and would be able to advocate for them in a similar manner.

It seems, therefore, that the nurses or the health professional closest to the patient is ideally placed to decide whether or not it might be appropriate to directly discuss donation with individual patients, but only if they know how to go about it, or whether information would be best provided by another method or person. However, it has been highlighted by the research from both the acute and palliative care settings that, for the reasons discussed within this chapter, they are at present likely to be extremely ambivalent about taking on this role. It seems, therefore, that in order for these attitudes to change and for nurses and other health care professionals to feel competent and confident in undertaking this role they will need to develop a greater awareness of the potential value of donation in palliative care, more knowledge of the donation process and the communication skills to sensitively initiate, if appropriate, conversation about this emotive subject. More education and support are therefore likely to be necessary.

Conclusion

In this chapter, we have established the potential contribution of non-heartbeating donors to the donotransplantation process and that there is limited research about organ and tissue donation outside the intensive care setting, even though these areas represent potentially valuable sources of tissues. The lack of agreement regarding criteria for death in non-heartbeating donors adds a layer of complexity to non-heartbeating organ donor policy, which remains a state of superficial and fragile consensus. The controversies about *irreversibility* and *time of death* in non-heartbeating policies are set to continue and will undoubtedly impact on the likelihood of increasing the donor pool for solid organ or tissue donation from non-heartbeating donors.

The relevant studies that we have examined suggest potential conflicts, difficulties and benefits that exist for patients, families and health professionals, and the differences that are presented when donation occurs outside the intensive care setting. All these areas require further investigation.

As with all qualitative research, the findings of the studies from the palliative care setting cannot be considered representative of all palliative care patients or health professionals. By providing accounts of the views of a small group of patients and professionals, they nevertheless highlight some of the complex issues that influence donation from within the palliative care environment and pinpoint the differences in the nature of the challenges faced by health care professionals working outside the intensive care setting.

Patients within intensive care are likely to be unconscious and thus unable to make their own choices about donation. Patients in other settings, such as palliative care, may well be able to and this is likely to influence the decision-making of professionals. Also, intensive care is a highly interventionist setting. Arguably, health care professionals practising in this environment may be less likely to experience the conflict of philosophies expressed by palliative care professionals, who aspire towards a 'non-medicalized' and 'natural' death for their patients. Given that the majority of terminally ill patients die outside the specialist palliative care environment, these issues may have relevance to, and thus be useful in informing, education initiatives and policy development of those working in clinical settings outside intensive care. From the evidence currently available we can put forward the following aspects of care for health professionals to consider:

- the contribution to be made to the donotransplantation by non-heartbeating donation and the need to establish viable donation policies;
- the need to be aware of the demand for donated tissue and the valuable contribution that it can make to a recipient's quality of life;
- the need to explore their own feelings and attitudes towards organ and tissue donation, because if it is to become part of their clinical role to inform patients and families of the choice, they need to feel knowledgeable, comfortable, supported and confident with the issue;
- while being sensitive to the delicacy of discussing donation it needs to be considered as a choice in end of life care;
- the evidence has shown that every patient will need a skilful assessment, by the health care team, to decide if, when and how they should receive donation information; thus, units will need to develop different methods of informing individuals about tissue donation, whether by direct discussion or indirectly, by having written information available for patients and families.

With an increasing necessity for patients outside intensive care to become donors, health care providers for patients who are potential donors should revise their procedures to facilitate organ preservation and retrieval. It seems vital therefore that those charged with the responsibility within health care organizations should examine their clinical practices and policies and consider initiatives, such as education programmes, that might help facilitate a greater commitment among health professionals towards the donation process. As yet, the evidence suggests there is a need to raise public and health care professionals' awareness regarding organ and tissue donation beyond the intensive care setting. We would recommend that health care professionals engage in open discussion regarding organ and tissue donation so as to formulate strategies to manage the challenges that have been highlighted within this chapter.

Notes

1   For the purpose of organ donation, non-heartbeating donation is defined as irreversible cessation of circulation, asystole, apnoea and unresponsiveness for a period of greater than two minutes. The preferred US term for non-

hearting donation is donation after cardiac death (DCD). Non-heartbeating donors can be divided into 4 categories:
Category 1 patients who are dead on arrival
Category 2 patients who have not responded to resuscitation
Category 3 awaiting death after withdrawal of life support
Category 4 brain dead patients in whom cardiac arrest occurs
Categories 1, 2 and 4 are referred to as uncontrolled donors. Category 3 do- nors are called controlled donors.
2   Donotransplantation includes the donation and transplantation process.

References

Ad Hoc Harvard Committee (1968) Report of Ad Hoc Committee of Harvard Medical School to examine definition of brain death. A definition of irre- versible coma, *Journal of the American Medical Association*, 205(6): 85–8.

Basu, P., Hazariwaza, K.M. and Chipman, M.L. (1989) Public attitudes toward donation of body parts particularly the eye, *Canadian Journal of Ophthalmol- ogy*, 24(5): 216–19.

Bridgare, S.A. and Oermann, M.H. (1991) Attitudes and knowledge of nurses re- garding organ procurement, *Heart and Lung*, 20: 20–4.

Bruera, E., Sweeney, C., Calder, K., Palmer, L. and Benisch-Tolley, S. (2001) Patient preferences versus physician perceptions of treatment decisions in cancer care, *Journal of Clinical Oncology*, 19(11): 2883–5.

Carey, I. and Forbes, K. (2003) The experiences of donor families in the hospice, *Palliative Medicine*, 17: 241–7.

Charmaz, K. (1980) *The Social Reality of Death: Death in Contemporary America*. Reading, MA: Addison-Wesley.

Clover, A., Browne, J., McErlain, P. and Vandenberg, B. (2004) Patient approaches to clinical conversations in the palliative care setting, *Journal of Advanced Nursing*, 48(4): 333–41.

Copp, G. (1999) *Facing Impending Death: Experiences of Patients and Their Nurses*. London: EMAP Healthcare.

Degner, L.F. and Sloane, J.A. (1992) Decision-making during serious illness: what role do patients really want to play? *Journal of Clinical Epidemiology*, 45: 941–50.

Doig, C. and Rocker, G. (2003) Retrieving organs from non-heart beating organ donors: a review of medical and ethical issues, *Canadian Journal of Anesthesia*, 50(10): 1069–76.

Enselberg, C.D. (1952) The dying human heart: electrocardiographic study of forty-three cases, with notes upon resuscitative attempts, *Archives of Internal Medicine*, 90: 15–29.

Feuer, D. (1998) Organ donation in palliative care, *European Journal of Palliative Care*, 5(1): 21–5.

Gallup (1993) *The American Public's Attitudes Toward Organ Donation and Trans-plantation*, www.transweb.org/reference/articles/gallup_survey/gallup_title.html (accessed 31 July 2006).

Garde, P.P. and Corbett, N.A. (1994) Organ donation: knowledge and attitudes of nursing and college students, *Journal of Transplant Coordination*, 4: 48–52.

Gore, S.M., Cable, D.J. and Holland, A.J. (1992) Organ donation from intensive care units in England and Wales: a two year confidential audit of deaths in intensive care, *British Medical Journal*, 304: 349–55.

Hughes, D. (2005) *'Evocative talk' in palliative care: discussing organ and tissue donation with hospice day care patients.* MSc thesis, University of Surrey, Guildford: UK.

Institute of Medicine (1997) *Non-Heart-Beating Organ Transplantation: Medical and Ethical Issues in Procurement.* Washington, DC: National Academy of Sciences.

Kennedy, I. (2003) Patients are experts in their own field, *British Medical Journal*, 326: 1276–7.

Kent, B. (2002) Psychosocial factors influencing nurses' involvement with organ and tissue donation, *International Journal of Nursing Studies*, 39: 429–40.

Kent, B. (2004) Protection behaviour: a phenomenon affecting organ and tissue donation in the 21st century? *International Journal of Nursing Studies*, 41(3): 273–84.

Kimber, R.M., Metcalfe, M.S., White, S.A. and Nicholson, M.L. (2001) Use of non-heart-beating donors in renal transplantation, *Postgraduate Medical Journal*, 77: 681–5.

Lawton, J. (2000) *The Dying Process: Patients' Experiences of Palliative Care.* London: Routledge.

Lewis, D.D. and Valerius, W. (1999) Organs from non-heart-beating donors: an answer to the organ shortage, *Critical Care Nurse*, 19: 70–4.

Madioni, F., Morales, M. and Michel, J. (1997) Body image and the impact of terminal disease, *European Journal of Palliative Care*, 4(5): 160–2.

Maguire, P. (1999) Improving communication with cancer patients, *European Journal of Cancer*, 35(10): 1415–22.

Mok, E. and Chiu, P.C. (2004) Nurse-patient relationships in palliative care, *Journal of Advanced Nursing*, 48(5): 475–85.

Murray, M., Miller, T., Fiset, V., O'Connor, A. and Jacobsen, M. (2004) Decision support: helping patients and families to find a balance at the end of life, *International Journal of Palliative Nursing*, 10(6): 270–7.

National Council for Hospice and Specialist Palliative Care Services (1995) *Specialist Palliative Care: A Statement of Definition.* Occasional paper 8. London: NCHSPCS.

National Institute for Clinical Excellence (2004) *Improving Supportive and Palliative Care for Adults with Cancer.* London: NICE.

Nekolaichuk, C.L. and Bruera, E. (1998) On the nature of hope in palliative care, *Journal of Palliative Care*, 14: 36–42.

Odell, J., Boyce, S. and Siddall, S. (1998) Tissue viability supplement. Tissue donation: the benefit of a positive approach, *Nursing Standard*, 13(3): 66–71.

O'Gorman, S.M. (1998) Death and dying in contemporary society: an evaluation of current attitudes and the rituals associated with death and dying and their relevance to recent understandings of health and healing, *Journal of Advanced Nursing*, 27(6): 1127–35.

Peters, D. and Sutcliffe, J. (1992) Organ donation: the hospice perspective, *Palliative Medicine*, 6: 212–16.

Quick, B. and Bastani, B. (1994) Prolonged asystolic hyperkalemic cardiac arrest with no neurologic sequelae, *Annals of Emergency Medicine*, 24: 305–11.

Rinopoche, S. (1995) *The Tibetan Book of Living and Dying*. London: Rider.

Robinson, G.C. (1912) A study with the electrocardiograph of the mode of death of the human heart, *Journal of Experimental Medicine*, 16: 291–302.

Rodstein, M. and Bornstein, M. (1970) Terminal ECG in the aged: electrocardiographic, pathological and clinical correlation, *Geriatrics*, 25: 91–100.

Ronaldson, S. and Devery, K. (2001) The experience of transition to palliative care services: perspectives of patients and nurses, *International Journal of Palliative Nursing*, 7(4): 171–7.

Spivey, M. (1998) *Organ/tissue donation within the palliative care setting*. BA honours dissertation, University of Luton, Luton: UK.

Sque, M. and Payne, S. (1994) Gift exchange theory: a critique in relation to organ transplantation, *Journal of Advanced Nursing*, 19: 45–51.

Sque, M. and Wells, J. (2004) Organ and tissue donation: helping patients and families to make choices, in S. Payne, J. Seymour and C. Ingleton (eds) *Palliative Care Nursing: Principles and Evidence for Practice*. Maidenhead: Open University Press.

Sque, M., Payne, S. and Vlachonikolis, L. (2000) Cadaveric donotransplantation: nurses' attitudes, knowledge and behaviour, *Social Science & Medicine*, 50: 541–52.

Thompson, S.C., Pitts, J.S. and Schwankovsky, C. (1993) Preferences for involvement in medical decision-making: situational and demographic influences, *Patient Education and Counselling*, 22: 133–40.

UK Transplant (2004) *Transplant Activity 2003*. Bristol: UK Transplant.

Walters, T. (1993) Modern death: taboo or not taboo? in D. Dickenson and M. Johnson (eds) *Death, Dying and Bereavement*. London: Sage.

Wells, J. (2004) *A Study to Investigate the Role and Value of Corneal Donation in the Palliative Care Setting*. Research report. University of Southampton, Southampton: UK.

Wells, J. and Sque, M. (2002) 'Living choice': the commitment to tissue donation in palliative care, *International Journal of Palliative Nursing*, 8(1): 22–7.

WHO (World Health Organization) (2002) *National Cancer Control Programmes: Policies and Managerial Guidelines*, 2nd edn. Geneva: WHO.

Willard, C. (2000) Cardiopulmonary resuscitation for palliative care patients: a discussion of ethical issues, *Palliative Medicine*, 14: 308–12.

Youngner, S., Arnold, R. and DeVita, M. (1999) When is 'dead'? *Hastings Center Report*, 29(6): 14–21.

8 Decisions about living kidney donation: a family and professional perspective

Patricia M. Franklin and Alison K. Crombie

Introduction[1]

Living renal donation is increasing due to excellent graft survival rates, a lack of growth in cadaveric donation and an increase in those waiting for a renal transplant. Indeed, in the USA the number of transplants from living renal donors has recently overtaken the number of transplants from deceased donors. Living renal donation involves complicated decision-making for donors, recipients and health professionals and is underpinned by legal constraints, national guidelines (see Appendix 1) and individual ethical, moral and familial attitudes.

The discussions within this chapter explore this decision-making with recourse to national and international data and two qualitative research studies, undertaken by each of the authors, in two large transplant centres in the UK (Franklin and Crombie 2003). To provide further insights into important core aspects of decision-making from the viewpoint of recipients, donors, non-donors, pre- and postoperatively, as well as biomedical decision-making, Franklin concentrated on psychological parameters, while Crombie explored the sociocultural perspectives, through an anthropological approach. Franklin and Crombie's fieldwork consisted of interviews with family members, interviews with transplant professionals (consultants, counsellors, nurses and other health professionals) and observation in transplant clinics, wards, dialysis units, and meetings between senior medical and multi-professional team members.

Background

Since the first human kidney transplant in 1954, solid organ transplantation now encompasses most organs in the body: heart, lung, kidneys, liver, pancreas, small and large intestine. Developments in surgical techniques and drugs to suppress bodily rejection have improved the success of and thus the requirement for all types of transplants. Because of the availability of an alternative treatment for kidney failure in the form of dialysis, the vast majority await a kidney transplant. Renal care, and particularly dialysis, has expanded very rapidly with the shortage of deceased organ donors, the return to dialysis of patients whose grafts have failed, and the increasing population of ageing individuals deemed medically unsuitable for transplantation (McMillian and Briggs 1995). Moreover there has been an increasing obligation on the health services to do everything possible to diagnose effectively and actively treat all renal problems, no matter what the limiting conditions may be (The Kidney Alliance 2001).

Donor organs in the UK are retrieved from two categories of donor, live and dead. A single kidney, as well as lobes of lung and liver can be donated while the donor is living; indeed living kidney donation is not new; the early renal transplants performed over 30 years ago before the use of criteria for brainstem death were, in the main, from living related donors. Over the past three decades donation from cadaveric sources, with death diagnosed either post-cardiac death, or using neurological criteria, has largely replaced living donation. The potential from cadaveric donations has not been realized in the way that transplant centres first envisaged, as highlighted by well-documented research (Gore *et al.* 1992; New *et al.* 1994; British Transplantation Society (BTS) 1995). Thus many centres worldwide have continued or renewed their interest in the use of living donors. In terms of discussions about meeting 'donor shortages', and improving transplant rates, live donation is now very high on the political agenda and indeed encouraging live donation is formal policy (BTS and The Renal Association 2000).

Living donation

Difficulties in procuring cadaveric organs for transplant are not the only reason for the expanding interest in the possibilities of achieving high levels of donation from live donors. It is argued that living donor transplantation can be planned more effectively and living kidney donations are associated with better results than cadaveric transplantation. In the case of kidney transplant, for example, the half-life of a cadaveric kidney (about 8 years) is significantly less than that for living donor kidneys (approximately 12 to 26 years) (Bradley and Nicholson 1999). Matches between family members are likely to produce better results, but living donor kidney transplants between genetically unrelated donors also tend to be more successful than cadaveric transplants with closer matching.

Nevertheless, live kidney donation poses physical and psychological 'risk' for the donor thus raising major ethical issues. Clinically the removal of an organ disadvantages rather than improves a donor's health. It exposes the donor to short-term risk of major surgery and the long-term consequences of living with a single kidney in the case of renal transplantation (Donnelly and Price 1997). Living donation challenges the basis of the Hippocratic principle, *primum nihil nocere* (first do no harm). Donnelly and Price found that although retrospective analysis indicates that the risks to the donor's health are minimal, few centres systematically review donor well-being. In addition, they illustrate that clinicians inevitably employ relatively subjective terms such as likely, probable, possible and moderate, to convey levels of risk. Therefore the basis for reassurance is not set against formal quantitatively-based criteria, and furthermore in biomedical practice levels of risk are often offset against the benefits of the procedure. For the live donor there are no physical benefits, but only the potential for psychological gain. In this respect psychiatric research over the years has reported contradictory findings. The early studies summarized by Franklin (2001: 708) 'questioned the fundamental willingness of relatives to make this type of sacrifice' (see also Chapter 3).

Family relationships are pivotal in live transplantation, however, the concept of the family is complex, and family structures have changed over time. Societal expectations that 'I am my brother's keeper' persist but are less relevant today; therefore, there is a need for relevant information from recent studies. A study by Schover *et al.* (1997) examined 167 donors with regard to the psychological aspects of the decision to donate, the impact of donation on family relationships, donors' reactions to graft failure and the overall satisfaction of donors. The study findings suggest that the majority of donors made the decision to donate with little ambivalence, expressed comfort with the choice at long-term follow-up and did not experience negative consequences regarding health or family relationships.

A study from the University of Minnesota with follow-up of 529 living donors concluded that donors scored higher than the general population with regard to quality of life issues. The research found the overall donor experience was stressful for 12 per cent, with donors more likely to say experiences were stressful if they had post-operative complications. If given the opportunity, only 4 per cent of the donors said that they would not donate again, and 9 per cent were unsure (Jacobs *et al.* 1998). Scandinavian studies reported similar findings. Westlie *et al.* (1990) reported that nearly 500 living donors in Norway were asked if they could turn the clock back, would they do the same again. Eight-three per cent said definitely 'yes', and another 11 per cent said 'probably yes'. In addition, many donors were deeply grateful for the opportunity to become a donor. Fehrman-Ekholm *et al.* (2000), reporting the Swedish experience, argued that less than 1 per cent of donors regretted the donation, although several experienced the first few months after the donation as troublesome from a physical perspective.

It is important to note that these studies were conducted by postal questionnaire, and such methodology lacks deep insight and can result in superficial responses that may not reflect the psychosocial ramifications that have been reported by other authors. Russell and Jacob (1993), commenting on existing research, noted that results indicated that while psychological side-effects have been reported, including depression and family conflict, these risks are generally under-emphasized. Furthermore, they postulated that by merely presenting the option of donation the individual is immediately placed under an unwarranted moral burden, and indeed potential donors are in a no-win situation. If potential donors say 'no', they are sure to regret the decision not to save a life, and if they say 'yes', they may regret not only the loss of an organ but also the lost opportunity to make up their minds without pressure. Therefore the act of consent is paramount. However, as others have noted, consent is dependent on a variety of complex factors and thus evades simple definitions.

Ellis and Bochner (1999) describe that informed consent is dependent as much on how we feel in conversations, our relationships with those giving information, and how information is given, as on the substantive content of what we are actually told. Informed consent is volatile, emotional and processual. People make up their minds, change, hold on, become confused, disagree, rationalize, blame, accept responsibility, reinterpret, misinterpret, do cost-benefit analyses and then act on what their emotions instruct them to do instead, or do not act, and simply do not know what to do. Thus the concept of autonomous consent is as ambiguous in living donation as has proved to be the case in other health-related settings.

As Price (1996) highlights, concerns have also been expressed about informed consent based on the way that donors make decisions. Simmons *et al.* (1977) and Fellner and Marshall (1970), in their studies among renal donors, have shown that, contrary to making a decision following adequate information-giving and assimilation of the risks to themselves, in the majority of cases the decision is made without deliberation and is immediate and spontaneous. As Price has argued, 'Informed consent is not legally or ethically suspect simply because decision-making is relatively instinctive and instantaneous' (1996: 112).

Decision to donate

Simmons *et al.* (1977) who were responsible for much of the early social research into the effects of live donation within families recognized that family pressure could be direct or subtle and also noted that pressure to donate could come from fear of family rejection or simply internal feelings of guilt. Kemph *et al.* (1969), Fellner and Marshall (1970) and Simmons *et al.* (1971)

reported that occasionally the 'black sheep' of the family offered to donate in an attempt to win approval and become reinstated within the family.

During the 1980s studies began to report more positive psychological findings. Thus the weight of evidence at that time led Surman (1989) to write that kidney donation had a favourable outcome for both donor and recipient, and the participation of living related donors in kidney transplantation was now widely accepted. Schover *et al.* (1997) concluded that the decision to donate was made with little ambivalence and that donors did not experience negative consequences regarding family relationships. More recently these findings were supported by a European study reported by Donnelly and Price (1997) who concluded that a very high percentage of donors knew very early on that they were going to donate and did not deliberate very long before reaching a decision. However, Russell and Jacob (1993) reported that by merely presenting the option the donor was immediately placed under an unwarranted moral burden, a no-win situation. Such a situation is graphically described by these authors as a sibling who felt like 'a fish on a hook'.

Parental donation decisions

Franklin and Crombie (2003) reported that all parent donors in Franklin's study stated that they had donated out of love as it was for them the natural thing to do. Indeed, one mother thought that any mother worth her salt would be prepared to die for her child. A father explained he had always felt some jealousy toward his wife because she had the experience of the birth of their son; he thought that donating would give him a similar bond with his child. All the parents in this study expressed surprise that any parent would refuse the chance to give this gift to their child.

Franklin and Crombie (2003) found similar responses from the mothers Franklin interviewed, but ambivalence from fathers. The mothers expressed altruistic motivation for donation. Franklin found the emphasis for these mothers was on the 'naturalness' of donating to a child, believing that giving a kidney was a natural extension of their role as a mother. In contrast, the decision-making experience was more complex for the fathers. The decision appears to have been based on a range of other, less powerful, motivating factors than the mothers' experiences of pregnancy and childbirth, which directly seemed to spur the mothers to donate. To illustrate, a female recipient's father suggested that he would have considered donation had the circumstances been life-threatening, but he indicated he would not have been anxious or eager to donate. He said he was very relieved that his wife was donating. Another father was reticent in his offer of a kidney to his daughter and appears to have responded to subtle situational pressure. He eventually volunteered to donate to his daughter only when his wife was unable so to do.

A difficult physical recovery and a long period of depression followed his apparent ambivalence before the operation.

Donation decisions by siblings

Sibling donation was found to be altruistic and uncomplicated in the majority of cases reported by Franklin and Crombie (2003). However, it was also reported that some sibling donors had different reasons for offering a kidney. For example, a sibling (female) stressed that she had donated to gain acceptance within the family as she had always been seen as the rebel, and all was forgiven when she offered to be a donor for her sister. This response was indicative of the early 'black sheep' findings of Simmons *et al.* (1977). Another sibling (male) did not wish to donate but went ahead anyway because he felt he couldn't have faced his parents if he had refused. Although he did not like his sister very much he felt it impossible to refuse once the request was made. He put it down to a sort of family and moral duty.

Franklin and Crombie's report (2003) supported the more complex decision-making for donor siblings although many of the siblings donated to alleviate the suffering and improve the quality of life for the recipient; donating out of familial duty and guilt was evident from the case studies.

Offered or approached?

All parents in Franklin and Crombie's (2003) studies offered as soon as the possibility of a transplant was suggested. The majority of siblings also offered before a request was made, however in some cases donors were asked to give, by one parent who acted as a go-between. Similar findings were reported by Franklin and Crombie (2003), who found that all the mothers offered. Mothers played an important role in sibling donation. There was often mediation and negotiation between family members as to the 'best fit' of a family member to assume the donor role. Parents, and particularly mothers, often took on the role of mediator and negotiator within the family. This role was not a 'neutral' one and often involved a clear view from the outset as to the likely donor. In some sibling donor cases, there was a process of subtle 'whittling down' of the array of possible family members who could donate a kidney.

The recipients' willingness to accept

Simmons *et al.* (1977) reported that although recipients did feel guilt about the gift that they could not reciprocate, most reported that they had no major problems with accepting the gift and that most recipients and donors reported that there were no major problems in their relationship a year post-transplant.

Franklin and Crombie (2003) also reported that many of the recipients accepted the offer of a transplant with alacrity but some recipients had misgivings. These occurred mainly in the cases of adolescents accepting from a parent, as well as in unusual sibling situations in which the recipient felt that the offer was an act of manipulation. The adolescents all expressed anxieties about the donation and possible future obligations to, and control by, the donor parent. Recipients also may have found it hard to refuse such an offer fearing donor rejection.

A female in Franklin and Crombie's (2003) report who received a kidney from her father stated that in many ways she would have liked to have refused but that would have caused so much conflict, and she needed her (family) support. She thought that afterwards she would have been expected to show 'eternal gratitude'. Her fears had been realized as she stated that her father never let her forget and that she always felt like the child who had to be obedient as she could never be grateful enough. A male recipient reported that his father continually phoned him at university to remind him to take care of himself and his father's kidney.

Adolescents often felt that they were not included in discussions about who their donor would be. One female recipient reported that she hated having her father's kidney inside her as she did not like him and she would not mind if she rejected the kidney as it would open the way for her to get one from a stranger. These findings of exclusion from decision-making in the case of adolescents were also reported by Franklin and Crombie (2003).

The decision not to donate

Franklin and Crombie's (2003) non-donor group reflects the findings of classical studies by Simmons *et al.* (1971, 1977), Simmons and Klein (1972) and Simmons (1983) in which data were collected from 186 non-donors. Crombie highlights how in several of her non-donation cases, potential donors did not donate as they did not consider there was a desperate need, perceiving their potential recipients as working and living relatively normal lives. Therefore, they appeared to reason, the situation for the potential recipient seemed not to be sufficiently serious to disrupt their own lives by donating a kidney.

In addition, as did Simmons *et al.* (1977) and Franklin (2001), Franklin and Crombie report conflict between the family of birth and the family of marriage. In several cases, the non-donors felt that the request to donate had come at the wrong time in their lives such as starting at university. It appeared that the choice not to donate a kidney disrupted family dynamics. It was not unusual to find resentment and disappointment among potential recipients, which was never openly discussed. The lack of open discussion between potential donors and recipients was a common thread that ran through many of the case histories reported. Moreover, in some cases, these issues may never be resolved.

Franklin and Crombie (2003) reported that there was resentment that the request had placed potential donors in an intolerable position and resulted in family conflict. For example, a recipient described how her mother was disappointed in the way that her brothers had not responded to what she saw as a family crisis. In her mother's view the situation was clear; her daughter's health took priority over her brothers' immediate needs. The recipient said that she remembered her mother standing up and being really angry, yelling and shouting at her brothers and insisting that one of them would donate.

Post-operative relationships

In support of Schover *et al.*'s (1997) findings Franklin (2001) reported that all donor and recipient siblings felt that their relationships were closer after the donation. The ongoing obligation, gratitude as defined by Fox and Swazey (1974, 1992), did not seem to have caused problems in the sibling group in her study and the donor and recipients seemed to have adjusted well to independent lives. One recipient reported that they always celebrated the date of the transplant with a thank-you meal together and it was not mentioned again for the rest of the year.

In contrast to Franklin (2001) and Schover *et al.* (1997), Franklin and Crombie's research supports the work of Fox and Swazey in that several of the donor and recipient sibling pairs discussed the difficulties of reciprocity. For example, they highlight the case of a female who received a kidney from one of her siblings who was close in age and geographic distance. However, the closeness to her sister and family served as a constant reminder, after the operation, of her debt to her sister. She stated that after the transplant it had been really difficult to row with her and very hard to say 'no'. The relationship clearly wasn't normal, they were no longer equals; she 'owed' her sister. She said she couldn't be herself and wasn't able to refuse looking after her kids, if she said, 'no' she felt mean. In the end she built up resentment and hated feeling like it, she felt the dynamics had really changed. Her mother's input had not helped, as she had interjected during a row: 'How could you, she gave you a kidney?'; which made the relationship worse. She said that people think if someone gives you a kidney that you are totally indebted to that person for the rest of your life, and she hadn't envisaged it. Nevertheless it must be noted that the principle of reciprocity did not override everything, payment was not expected and although recipients talked of having a debt of gratitude, this was not always an uncomfortable debt.

In both Franklin and Crombie's (2003) studies the parent to adolescent child relationship were not so straightforward and in several cases did mirror the findings reported by Fox and Swazey with regard to donor intrusion into recipients' lifestyles and the recipient being burdened by an indebtedness that could never be repaid. Such feelings had caused psychological distress and damaged relationships as Fox and Swazey (1992) predicted. The level of psychological distress reported in Franklin's study was such that two subjects stated that a cadaveric graft might have been preferable. These findings are in sharp contrast to the conclusions reported by Baines *et al.* (2001) who found that parent to child donation did not appear to have any detrimental effects on family dynamics. However, the children in this study were younger and it may be that the adolescent to parent conflict reported by Franklin and Crombie was underpinned by the usual difficulties experienced in most child-parent relationships during adolescence. Donation and transplantation appear to have enhanced such conflict, which in some cases had not been resolved.

A further component in the ramifications of live donation is the initial approach and subsequent support from biomedical and health care professionals. An aspect of Crombie's (1997) research explored decision-making in live donation from the perspective of senior medical clinicians involved in this process.

Biomedical decision-making in living donation

There is a dearth of research which relates to key professionals involved in supporting and making decisions about living donation. Nevertheless there is a body of sociological and anthropological literature that argues for biomedicine to be explored as a cultural system. As Scheper-Hughes and Lock (1987), Good (1990) and Casper and Koenig (1996) have highlighted, it is important to dispute the concept that biomedicine, because it is so highly developed scientifically and technologically, is not imprinted with cultural beliefs and values. Many scientific notions have been contested and shown to be the product of mystification in which the social relations producing scientific knowledge are disguised (Latour and Woolgar 1979; Gilbert and Mulkay 1984; Casper and Koenig 1996). That is, they have highlighted what scientists actually do, rather than focusing solely on structures, interests, or particular individuals or institutions. These routine, everyday practices are integral to changes in the way in which the body and its materials are conceptualized. Therefore, in developing an understanding of decision-making among clinicians in relation to living kidney donation it is necessary to acknowledge broader sets of rhetorically 'rational' biomedical knowledge, but also to see this knowledge as invariably historically and culturally situated.

Attitudes among practitioners to child to parent donation

Although many medical practitioners embrace the concept of living donation as a realistic treatment option for the patient and family, it appears that in some cases individual social and cultural criteria influence decisions in relation to donation (Crombie 1997). Thus reference to formal medical criteria appeared to covertly mask personal attitudes, which on occasions influenced decision-making to exclude some donors rather than others.

Research has found differences in attitudes and in practice to accepting particular individuals in certain kinship relationships as donors (Crombie 1997). The research also provided detailed insight into the differing attitudes and practice between clinicians. These differences observed in one transplant centre may help to explain the disparity in the numbers of transplants performed nationally.

For example, while most clinicians at the transplant centre agreed that parents, siblings, offspring and other relatives should all be considered as donors in principle, it became apparent through the process of observation over time that some clinicians were reluctant to transplant from offspring to parent. For example, during a review meeting the case of a 60-year-old man who had been on dialysis with one failed cadaveric transplant was raised. His 23-year-old daughter wished to donate one of her kidneys to her father. A physician suggested that she should be tested for compatibility; however in contrast his colleague was clear that the man should wait until a cadaveric transplant became available. Following up this decision in a later conversation the colleague explained that he did not try and put people off but he would rather an older rather than a younger donor because the donor still had the rest of their life to get through with only one kidney, which in the case of a young donor may be some 50 years. Yet the explanation is not particularly logical if live donation is promoted as a safe procedure, and younger siblings do donate to each other.

This appears different from the ethical issues that relate to minors who have become almost formally excluded from donating non-regenerative tissue, even though many of the earliest successful living renal transplants, in the 1950s and early 1960s, involved minor donors. Recent guidelines from the British Transplant Society and the Renal Association state that: 'Individuals under the age of eighteen years should rarely, if ever, be considered as potential living kidney donors' (British Transplant Society and The Renal Association 2000: 13). In any case, this recommendation appears to follow, in a relatively standard way, often legally enforced prohibitions and restrictions on other actions of 'minors'.

In contrast, older donors may also be considered problematic as the chances of health problems increase with age compounding the risks to the donor. An exchange in a clinic between a medical colleague and a young female patient who was on dialysis illustrates these issues. The patient raised the possibility of her father in his late 60s donating his kidney. The clinician explained that there was a high chance that the kidney would not do as well as a kidney from a younger donor and suggested that she might be off dialysis for a while but the kidney would possibly fail and then she would come back on dialysis, but with increased antibodies (these form following a failed transplant and make matching of successive transplants more difficult). He did not encourage her to further explore the option. Thus it appears that although in biomedical terms the younger donor might be a better option for the patient there is an obvious reluctance by clinicians to consider the do-nation from child to parents, and also there appears to be reluctance by some clinicians to consider older donors.

Furthermore this work illustrates that in some cases there was reluctance to consider donors with dependants. This view of not encouraging donors with dependants was demonstrated in an outpatient's clinic consultation where a patient raised the issue of his sister with young children wanting to donate. The clinician was ambivalent and wary because of the dependants. He said that he may not stop the donation but he would be concerned to know who would look after the children; he reiterated that it was a major operation, not without risk.

These issues are similar to the attitudes that were collated by the Eurotold project that found considerable reluctance among clinicians in response to a number of case study scenarios (Donnelly and Price 1997). It has been noted by Simmons (1983) that to deny the donor the right to donate could do psychological harm. Clinicians were not unaware of the difficulties involved in the gatekeeping position that is inevitably required of them (Crombie 1997). One of the clinicians noted that they had to be careful and aware as professionals not to impose their values on other people's sense of what is and what is not acceptable and that ultimately people have to make their own decisions.

Attitudes to borderline donors

Before 2000 few UK transplant centres systematically reviewed donor well-being and long-term donor follow-up was not carried out. Therefore the basis for reassurance to donors was not set against formal criteria. The decision as to who constitutes a suitable donor is not straightforward and is based on agreed guidelines only. There are varied opinions as to the acceptability of borderline cases; for example, blood pressure at the upper limit of normal range, renal function at the lower limit of normal range. The position of older donors (interpreted by some as being over 50 or 55 years of age and in others as over 60 or 65), and donors with multiple renal arteries (which makes the surgery more complex), led to different decisions. For example, mild hypertension (raised blood pressure) may exclude a donor for one clinician whereas this may be acceptable for a colleague. Clinicians each had their own interpretation of levels of risk, based on their unique experience and the paucity of scientific evidence.

Crombie argues that in most centres the initiative to introduce the subject of live donation remains with the physicians, but ultimate responsibility rests with the surgeons. The surgeon has ultimately to take the responsibility and carry out the operation. Even though there are national guidelines on what constitutes a borderline case in relation to living donation, it is still left to individual clinicians to decide precisely who or what constitutes such a case, or exactly in what ways the donor and their family should have a role in decision-making.

Conclusion

Franklin's and Crombie's research highlighted a number of concerns that health professionals working in the field of living donation need to be aware of. The studies suggest that the decision to donate is immediate and altruistic for most parents although some fathers expressed a degree of ambivalence. The decision to donate is reported to be more difficult and complex for siblings and may in some cases lead to difficulties and conflict between family of birth and family of marriage. Reciprocity and feelings of obligation did not appear to cause relationship difficulties for the majority of siblings although difficulties were reported by some. Feelings of obligation were more readily reported in parent to adolescent child recipient cases and had on occasions led to psychological distress and social-familial alienation. These complexities should be given greater priority within transplant programmes and professional care provided to ensure confidential pre-surgery donor and recipient advocacy.

Crombie found that despite their different ways of operating, clinicians converge in an approach to live donation which is at times 'idiosyncratic', but is nonetheless considered and sensitive. Thus what appears to be a robust, formal and direct biomedical approach to living kidney donation by those professionally involved in the process, has within it many different social and cultural sets of assumptions which impact on the practice of transplantation. Living kidney donation involves a complex social transaction in which powerful cultural beliefs are embedded in the process, and not just, as might be expected, among family members but also among the professional staff managing the process.

Notes

1   It may be helpful to readers to refer to Appendix 1, which explains the law in UK with regard to donations from living persons.

References

Baines, L.S., Beattie, T.J., Murphy, A.V. and Jindal, R.M. (2001) Relationship between donors and paediatric recipients of kidney transplant: a psychosocial study, *Transplantation Proceedings*, 33: 1897–9.

Bradley, A. and Nicholson, M. (1999) Renal transplantation from living donors should be seriously considered to help overcome the shortfall in organs, *British Medical Journal*, 318: 409–10.

British Transplantation Society (1995) *Report of the British Transplantation Society on Organ Donation*. London: Novartis.

British Transplantation Society and The Renal Association Working Party (2000) *United Kingdom Guidelines for Living Donor Kidney Transplantation*. London: Novartis.

Casper, M.J. and Koenig, B.A. (1996) Reconfiguring nature and culture: intersections of medical anthropology and technosciences, *Medical Anthropology Quarterly*, 10: 523–36.

Crombie, A. (1997) *Medical decision-making in live donation*. MSc thesis, University of Surrey, Guildford: UK.

Donnelly, P. and Price, D. (1997) *Questioning Attitudes to Living Donor Transplantation: European Multicentre Study, Transplantation of Organs from Living Donors Ethical and Legal Dimensions*. Leicester: The Project Management Group.

Ellis, C. and Bochner, A. (1999) Bringing emotion and personal narrative into medical social science, *Health*, 3: 229–37.

Fehrman-Ekholm, I., Brink, B., Ericsson, C., Elinder, C.G., Duner, F. and Lundgren, G. (2000) Kidney donors don't regret: follow-up of 370 donors in Stockholm since 1964, *Transplantation*, 69(10): 2067–71.

Fellner, C.H. and Marshall, J.R. (1970) The myth of informed consent, *American Journal of Psychiatry*, 126: 1245–51.

Fox, R.C. and Swazey, J.P. (1974) *The Courage to Fail: A Social View of Organ Transplants and Dialysis*. Chicago: University of Chicago Press.

Fox, R.C. and Swazey, J.P. (1992) *Spare Parts*. Oxford: Oxford University Press.

Franklin, P. (2001) Psychological aspects of kidney transplantation and organ donation, in P. Morris (ed.) *Kidney Transplantation: Principles and Practice*, 5th edn. Philadelphia, PA: W.B. Saunders.

Franklin, P.M. and Crombie, A.K. (2003) Live related renal transplantation: psychological, social, and cultural issues, *Transplantation*, 76(8): 1247–52.

Gilbert, N.G. and Mulkay, M. (1984) *Opening Pandora's Box: A Sociological Analysis of Scientist Discourse*. Cambridge: Cambridge University Press.

Good, B. (1990) *Medicine, Rationality and Experience: An Anthropological Perspective.* Cambridge: Cambridge University Press.

Gore, S.M., Cable, D.J. and Holland, A.J. (1992) Organ donation from intensive care units in England and Wales: a two year confidential audit of deaths in intensive care, *British Medical Journal*, 304: 349–55.

Jacobs, C., Johnson, E., Anderson, K. *et al.* (1998) Kidney transplants from living donors: how donation affects family dynamics, *Advanced Renal Therapy*, 5: 89.

Kemph, J.P., Bermann, E.A. and Coppolillo, H.P. (1969) Kidney transplants and shifts in family dynamics, *American Journal Psychiatry*, 125: 39–44.

Latour, B. and Woolgar, S. (1979) *Laboratory Life: The Social Construction of Scientific Facts*. Beverly Hills, CA: Sage.

McMillian, M.A. and Briggs, J.D. (1995) Survey of patient selection for cadaveric renal transplantation in the UK, *Nephrology Dialysis Transplantation*, 99: 855–8.

New, W., Solomon, M., Dingwell, R. and McHale, J. (1994) *A Question of Give and Take: Improving the Supply of Donor Organs for Transplantation*. London: Kings Fund Institute.

Price, D.P.T. (1996) The voluntarism and informedness of living donors, in D.P.T. Price and H. Akveld (eds) *Living Organ Donation in the Nineties: European Medico-legal Perspectives*. Leicester: European Commission.

Russell, S. and Jacob, R. (1993) Living-related organ donation: the donor's dilemma, *Patient Education and counselling*, 21(6): 89–99.

Scheper-Hughes, N. and Lock, M. (1987) The mindful body: a prolegmenon to future work in medical anthropology, *Medical Anthropology Quarterly*, 1(1): 6–41.

Schover, L., Streem, S.B., Boprai, N., Duriak, K. and Novick, A.C. (1997) The psychosocial impact of donating a kidney: long term follow up from a urology based centre, *The Journal of Urology*, 157(5): 1596–601.

Simmons, R.G. (1983) Long term reactions of renal recipients and donors, in N.B. Levy (ed.) *Psychonephrology*. New York: Plenum.

Simmons, R.G. and Klein, S.D. (1972) The search for kidney donors, *The American Journal of Psychiatry*, 129: 687–92.

Simmons, R.G., Hickley, K. and Kjellstrand, C. (1971) Donors and non-donors: the role of the family and the physician in kidney transplantation, *Seminars in Psychiatry*, 3(9): 102–15.

Simmons, R.G., Klein, G.S. and Simmons, R.I. (1977) *Gift of Life: The Effect of Organ Transplantation on Individual, Family and Societal Dynamic*. New York: Wiley.

Surman, O.S. (1989) Psychiatric aspects of organ transplantation, *American Medical Journal of Psychiatry*, 146: 972–82.

The Kidney Alliance (2001) *End Stage Renal Failure: A Framework for Planning and Services Delivery. Towards Equity and Excellence in Renal Services*. London: The Kidney Alliance.

Westlie, L., Talseth, T., Fauchald, P., Jakobsen, A. and Flatmark, A. (1990) A quality of life in living donors, *Kidney International*, 37: 124.

9 Xenotransplantation and the post-human future

Mary Murray

> *When they see the half-pig man ... The brute beasts will be heard to speak ...*
> (Nostradamus, cited in Mekdeci 1997)

Introduction

Xeno is the Greek for strange or foreign. Xenotransplantation involves any procedure involving the transplantation, implantation or infusion of cells, tissues or organs from non-human animals into the human body. Xenotransplantation was first described in Indian mythology. According to a Sanskrit text from the twelfth century BC the Indian gods Shiva and Parvati had a child, Ganesha, who was born a giant. Shiva beheaded Ganesha and returned him to life with an elephant's head (Deschamps *et al.* 2005). Human animal hybrids however long predate this mythological account of xenotransplantation. Combinations of human and non-human animal, humanimal, figure in Greek mythology. The Esfinge for example combined the head of a woman with the body of a winged lion. The Minotaur, offspring resulting from the sexual union of a woman and a bull, combined the body of a bull and the head of a man. Celtic mythology is also populated with deities who have animal features such as antlers or horns (Mac Cana 1984). The Egyptian pantheon is littered with gods that have ram's, bull's, cow's, lion's, cat's, bird's, hippopotamus', crocodile's and frog's heads. The more well known of such Egyptian figures is probably Anubis, who was connected to the funerary world as the god of mummification, and a conductor of the dead. Anubis combined a human body with the head of a jackal (Germond 2001).

Humanimals have also figured prominently in art and literature. Humananimal hybrids are depicted in the art of prehistoric caves and rock shelters. The great painted caves at Lascaux, Chauvet, Pech Merle and Altamira include depictions of supernatural and chimeral beings including humanimals such as the Lascaux bird man and the Chauvet bison man and lion woman (Hancock 2005). Medieval and modern painters including Hieronymous

Bosch in the fifteenth century, Goya and Blake in the eighteenth and nineteenth centuries, and twentieth-century surrealists including, Salvador Dali, have depicted fantastic monsters and chimeras, including humanimals, in their art. Contemporarily, the hybrid creatures of the artist Patricia Piccinini (2006) interweave human and animal worlds through a combination of the ultra-modern and the primordial.

One of the most popular literary forms in medieval Europe, the Bestiaries, included a range of human animal hybrids. They included the Sphinx, a human-headed lion, the Cynocephalus, a dog-headed human (Salisbury 1994) and the Monster of Cracow, a composite of human, ape, dog, toad, and cat (Shildrick 2002). Ostensibly 'scientific' when science included attempts to understand all truth, especially metaphysical truth, the Bestiaries were designed as allegories to teach humans lessons and tell them how to behave (Salisbury 1994). In this respect, 'monstrous births' were commonly explained as the progeny of unnatural intercourse between animals and humans (Salisbury 1994). Human-animal hybrids and shape shifters such as Dracula and the werewolf that populated the Gothic imagination continue to engage the popular imagination today, as do an array of human-animal hybrids found in contemporary popular culture, fantasy and science fiction writing and film. These include *The Fly*, the film interpretation of Kafka's (1961) *Metamorphosis*, as well as Tolkien's (1995) *The Lord of the Rings* and C.S. Lewis' (1993) *The Lion, the Witch and The Wardrobe*, both of which have been adapted for film.

Human-animal hybrids are however no longer the sole preserve of mythological, surreal and Gothic imaginations. Nor are human-animal hybrids confined to science fiction. Science itself is activating archaic and ancient humanimal archetypes and mythological monsters. In recent years science has produced, for example, Dolly the cloned sheep, the mouse with a human ear grafted onto its back and genetically engineered animals such as rabbits and cows carrying human genes. Genetically engineered pigs, carrying human genes, have also been produced for the purposes of xenotransplantion. These pigs are an outcome of the long history of xenotransplantation, a technology that has developed alongside xenotransfusions and xenografts.

History of xenotransplantation

Deschamps *et al.* (2005) have documented the history of xenotransplantation. At the beginning of the sixteenth century an Iranian surgeon reported a xenograft of dog bone as a replacement for human bone. In the seventeenth century, bone from a dog's skull was used to repair a human skull. There were documented cases of xenografts from human to animal and from animal to animal during the eighteenth century and from animal to human in the ninteenth century (Keys 1973; Kuss and Bourget 1992; Deschamps *et al.*

2005). Perhaps some of the most startling xenografts are those connected to sexual reproductive systems of different species. They were seen as a means of revitalization and renewal. In 1889 a French-American doctor injected himself with extract of crushed guinea pig and dog testicle (Dartigues 1925; Deschamps *et al.* 2005). In 1920 slices of chimpanzee testicle were placed in a human scrotum (Voronoff 1924). Ovaries from female apes have also been used for the treatment of menopause (Champsaur 1929). Ovaries from a female human have been transplanted into a female chimp (Champsaur 1929). The chimp was then inseminated with human sperm, but no pregnancy occurred. There are records too of organ xenografts from the early twentieth century. In 1905 slices of rabbit kidney were put into the kidney of a child (Deschamps *et al.* 2005). In 1906 pig kidney was attached to the bend of a middle-aged woman's elbow, and a goat kidney was transplanted to the elbow bend of a 50-year-old woman. A few years later a macaque kidney was transplanted to a young woman and a few years after that a kidney from a monkey was transplanted to the arm of a young girl (Kuss and Bourget 1992; Deschamps *et al.* 2005). In 1923 a lamb's kidney was transplanted to a man who had been poisoned with mercury (Neuhof 1923). A number of these kidney recipients died while others had to have the xenograft removed.

The first documented case of xenotransfusion occurred in 1667 when lamb's blood was given to a young man (Farr 1980; Deschamps *et al.* 2005). This was followed by the transfusion of calf's blood to a 34-year-old man in an attempt to cure him of madness. There were more recorded accounts of xenotransfusions later in the seventeenth century and during the nineteenth century. One of the objectives of xenotransfusion was to try and determine what, if any, qualities could be passed on to humans from animal blood. In a communication with the Royal Society, a seventeenth-century recipient of lamb's blood noted, humorously, 'Sheep's blood possesses a symbolic relationship with the blood of Christ, since Christ is the Lamb of God' (Deschamps *et al.* 2005: 92).

Following a gap of some 40 years, xenotransplantation began again in the 1960s. During this decade kidneys from a variety of primates were transplanted into humans, all of whom subsequently died. The resumption of xenotransplantation included heart transplantation. In 1963 the heart from a chimpanzee called Bino was transplanted into a man in his late 60s (Deschamps *et al.* 2005). In 1968 a sheep's heart was transplanted into a middle-aged man and in 1977, Dr Christian Barnard, who had performed the first human-to-human heart transplantation, transplanted a baboon's heart to a 25-year-old woman and a chimpanzee's heart to a 60-year-old man (Deschamps *et al.* 2005). In 1984 'Baby Fae' received a baboon's heart. All of the animal organ recipients died. The failure of these and earlier experiments led to a *de facto* moratorium for nearly a decade. Rejection of the animal organ by the human immune system was identified as a major obstacle that needed to be overcome.

Xenotransplantation resumed in the 1990s with the development of new immunosuppressive agents. Although primates were used as donors in the 1990s they are no longer considered as potential 'donors' because of risks of infectious disease transmission (Deschamps *et al.* 2005). In comparison to other species, the rate of reproduction among primates is low, their population numbers are low and international trade in chimpanzees is banned. While primates are used in other forms of medical and scientific research, currently there is, effectively, a worldwide moratorium preventing the use of primates for xenotransplantation (O'Neill 2006).

Today, pigs are the preferred species for xenotransplantation. Unlike primates, pigs are genetically and immunologically more distant from humans (Deschamps *et al.* 2005). However, pigs and humans are anatomically and physiologically quite similar. Pigs also reproduce rapidly. Under ideal conditions it is possible for a sow to have seven million descendants in a decade (Caspari 2003). Moreover, since the 1990s, transgenic pigs carrying human genes have been produced. The purpose of genetically engineering pigs in this way is to try and help prevent rejection of animal organs by the human immune system (Somerville 2000; Deschamps *et al.* 2005; O'Neill 2006).

However, the possibility of porcine endogenous retroviruses (PERVs) infecting human cells has been identified. Fears about zoonosis, the transmission of disease from animals to humans, have been animated in recent times by AIDS, 'mad cow disease' and 'bird flu', all of which have involved animal to human infection. While not wanting to minimize the dangers of cross-species infection, in the discussion that follows I want to think about fears of xenozoonosis in terms of what it may suggest about our sense of ourselves as humans and our relationship with other species.

To do this I will begin by outlining the findings of some anthropological and sociological research concerning the experiential impact of human to human organ transplantation among organ recipients. I will then think about fears of xenozoonosis in terms of boundaries that have been drawn between humans and other species, and link a reading of such anxieties to discourses of 'otherness'. This will be connected to Donna Haraway's observations that 'Immune system discourse is about the constraint and possibility for engaging in a world full of "difference", replete with non-self' (Haraway 1991: 214). It will also be linked to changing conceptions of the body, the skin and the self, as well as negative human characteristics that are projected onto animals, in particular, the pig.

Experiential impact of human to human organ transplantation

Accounts of organ recipients living in fear of perceived independent or animate qualities of their new organs might sound like an urban myth, or perhaps a scenario from science fiction. However, research indicates human to human organ transplantation can indeed be personally transformative, significantly altering recipients' definitions of themselves. Despite discouragement from medical professionals, organ recipients have reported a change in their sense of who they are to include assumed qualities of the organ donor (Sharpe 1995). While human organs tend to be reified by transplant professionals as bits of flesh, filters, pumps and muscles, organ recipients have reported profound effects on the transformation of identity according to the symbolic weight of the organ. In western society body organs such as lungs and hearts have powerful metaphoric significance linked to what it means to be human and alive. While lungs can symbolize the breath of life, hearts can symbolize passion and love, and may be perceived as seats of the soul or self. While organ recipients may fear the independent or animate qualities of donated organs, recipients may view such qualities more positively: where a young man's lungs have been received for example, recipients may refer to positive feelings such as strength and youth. Where a woman's heart has been received, the quality of gentleness may be remarked upon (Sharpe 1995). Research data therefore indicates that a reconstruction or transformation of one's sense of self to include a sense of the essence of the dead organ donor can be experienced. Indeed, while donors are encouraged to regard their organs as 'gifts', research indicates that the family of a dead donor may believe that their relative can in some way live on in another person's body (Sharpe 1995).

Organ recipients may experience themselves as amalgams of 'self' and 'other'. The idea of closed bodily integrity, and the associated modernist view that identity is located within an individual bounded self with a unified identity and a unique personality is therefore challenged by human to human organ transplantation (Lock 1995). Whereas the Cartesian view of identity is in terms of the *cogito* ego, human to human organ transplantation also shows that embodiment is significant to definitions of identity because it is through the body that we experience the world. If recipients of human organs can experience a change in the sense of themselves, what might be the experiential impact of receiving an animal organ? Transplant and psychological specialists may be particularly concerned to dissuade animal organ recipients from identification with the 'donor' or their species. Whereas a human organ may be thought of as a 'gift', transplant and psychological specialists may be even more inclined to emphasize a reified and commodified view of animal organs. Even so, perceiving animal organs in this way may occur precisely *because* xenotransplantation impacts upon how we understand ourselves, human society and culture. Some of the concern about transplanting animal organs into humans might be connected to an intuition, embedded, perhaps, in fears of xenozoonosis, that boundaries we have drawn between humans and the animal 'other' are breached, and that this calls into question the human, and perhaps the humane, in our 'nature'.

'Other' boundaries and breaches

The conceptual placing of animals, fixing them in a series of abstract spaces and distinguishing clean animals from unclean, can be traced back to pre-Neolithic totemic societies and the biblical classifications of different beasts in the ancient and medieval great chain of being (Philo and Wilbert 2000). Contemporarily, part of the 'imaginative geography' (Said 1978) of modernity has involved a positioning of animals (them) in relation to humans (us) in a way that combines geographical othering with conceptual othering. Animals are fixed in places and spaces that are different to the places and spaces that humans are located in. Animals and humans have also been perceived as having particular character traits (a point to which I will return later). This combination of geographical and conceptual othering has, in western society, involved non-domesticated animals becoming more distanced from humans. While it may be acceptable for some species to live in close proximity to humans, it is not acceptable for all species. It is acceptable for pets or 'companion animals' such as cats and dogs to live in towns and cities with humans in their dwelling places. The countryside however is seen as the proper place for farmed animals such as cows, sheep and pigs (Philo and Wilbert 2000). Whereas in the medieval European countryside livestock animals such as sheep, cows and pigs might share the actual dwelling places of the rural peasantry, in the modern European countryside such practices are no longer acceptable.

Anthropologist Mary Douglas has written a good deal on societal ideas about pollution (Douglas 1978). She points out that once pathogenicity and hygiene are abstracted from it, 'dirt' is simply 'matter out of place'. The idea of matter being out of place implies a set of ordered relations and a violation of such relations. The emergent product, dirt, links to symbolic ideas regarding pollution and purity that are embedded in relationships normally held in by rituals of separation. Regarding animals Douglas observes that '. . . in general the underlying principle of cleanness in animals is that they should conform fully to their class' (1978: 53).

The idea of pollution and nonconformity to class is, it can be argued, inextricably linked to our ideas about being 'in place' and 'out of place'.

LIVERPOOL JOHN MOORES UNIVERSITY
LEARNING SERVICES

Relating this to relations between humans and other animals, Jones (2000) has observed that relationships between humans and other species are embedded in the spatial organization of the planet. Geographies of place and space shape the human encounter with other species. A special taxonomy of animals exists. This uses classifications such as domestic pets, farm animals, zoo animals, laboratory animals and wild animals. With the exception of domestic pets and companion animals, the place and space of non-human animals is usually different and 'other' to the space and place of humans. In terms of farm animals such as cows and sheep, modern agricultural practices are such that it is unusual for them to get 'out of place'. From birth to death, the lives of such animals are spatially ordered and controlled. Relating such considerations to xenotransplantation, it would seem that admitted into the 'sacred' space of the human body and the societal space that it occupies, 'profane' animals appear to slip out of place. In so doing they may confound our ideas of sacredness with uncleanness and call into question the boundaries that we have drawn between humans and other animals.

We might read the fears of xenozoonosis that accompany the possibility of such boundary transgressions as a discourse of 'otherness' and alterity. Such discourses have been widespread in western society. They have included classism, racism, anti-feminism, heterosexism and nationalism. These discourses have been pervasive in the delineation and designation of social space and the formation of western subjectivity. Social scientists and historians have detailed ways in which state and empire in the West have been constructed *in* and *through* relations and discourses of class, race and gender domination (Corrigan and Sayer 1987; Haraway 1989; Murray 1995). These relations and institutions have been mapped onto social space defining, for example, borders of nation states, geographies of class and race, and the boundaries of public (male) and private (female) arenas. The formation of subjectivity in the West has also been inextricably linked to discourses of 'otherness', with identity being narrated through discourses that include nationality, masculinity and femininity, ethnicity and class allegiance.

'Other' bodies: speciesism and immune system discourse

The discourse of *species* is also firmly embedded in western society. As a discourse of 'otherness' and alterity, the discourse of species has been pervasive in the carving up of social space. Moreover, in the West the 'animal' has been part of a cultural history that goes back thousands of years. Cary Wolfe observes that 'It is this pervasiveness of the discourse of species that has made the *institution* of speciesism fundamental ... to the formation of western subjectivity and sociality' (2003: 6). Narratives of 'what it means to be human' have been constructed in and through ideas about animality. The institution of speciesism relies on an assumption that to be fully human we need to sacrifice the 'animal' and the animalistic (Wolfe 2003: 6) within us and among us. Our understanding of human society, historically and cross-culturally, has also been predicated upon the inclusion and exclusion of different species.

The discourse and institution of speciesism defines and privileges alterity not simply between human and non-human animals, but also within the human species: African and Aboriginal peoples, for example, were once thought of as not fully human and treated accordingly. The discourse and institution of speciesism also defines and privileges 'otherness' between non-human animals. Europeans may refuse to eat a pet dog but nevertheless enjoy roast cow. Other societies may have no qualms about eating dogs, while others may refuse to eat cow because of religious prohibitions.

'Difference' might be defined by a number of interrelated discourses within the discursive field such as nationalism, colonialism and racism. In relation to 'difference' between animals, I would suggest that speciesism is aided and abetted by immune system discourse. Haraway (1991) has written about the constitutions of self and other in immune system discourse. While not wanting to deny the clinical significance of the immune system she sees the immune system as an 'iconic mythic object' in which there is an intimate interweaving of 'Myth, laboratory and clinic' (1991: 205). The immune system 'is an elaborate icon for principle systems of symbolic and material "difference" in late capitalism. Pre-eminently a 20th century object, the immune system is a map drawn to guide recognition and misrecognition of self and other in the dialectics of Western biopolitics. That is, the immune system is a plan for meaningful action to construct and maintain the boundaries for what may count as self and other ...' (1991: 204). The immune system is imaged as a battlefield and the self as a defended stronghold. It provides a diagram of relationships and '... a guide for action in the face of questions about the boundaries of the self ...' (1991: 214).

Simians occupy the borderlands between nature and culture (Haraway 1989). Such ambiguity is perhaps underscored by the immunological similarity of other primates to humans. It is an ambiguity that is also played out in the way in which primates are and are not used in medical and scientific research. Speciesism has been used to justify the use of primates in a range of psychological and medical research such as investigations into maternal deprivation and treatment for AIDS. It is then the difference and similarity of other primates to humans that has been deemed a prerequisite for their use in many forms of research. On the other hand, speciesism has been used to try and exclude and protect primates from being subject to xenotransplantation. Primates such as chimps and baboons are closer to humans on the evolutionary scale than other species. They are highly intelligent, look like humans in significant ways, and have complex social and kinship organization. Such anthropocentric considerations, combined with low rates of reproduction, limited supply and a propensity to carry disease that can be passed on to humans (O'Neill 2006) makes primates unlikely xenotransplant 'donors'.

To try and prevent the rejection of the 'alien' animal organ by the human recipient, genetically engineered pigs, where human genes are introduced into the porcine foetus, have been developed. However, fears about xeno-zoonosis remain. This could mean that pig genes might need to be manipulated to a greater extent than previously thought necessary, to the extent that the resulting animal would not be recognized as a pig (O'Neill 2006). If a genetically modified pig were no longer recognized as a pig, bearing in mind the impact that human to human organ transplantation can have on identity, how might xenotransplantation affect an organ recipient's sense of their humanness? To what extent might the recipient of a major animal organ, such as a heart, experience anxieties connected to ideas about 'the beast within'? These kinds of fears, articulating a discourse of animality and alterity, may already be embedded in our fears about xenozoonosis.

Skin deep and under my skin

The transplantation of animal tissue into the human body is a long established practice. Pig valves can be used to replace human heart valves and to provide easy venous access for people receiving kidney dialysis. Such practices are widespread and do not appear to raise the same kinds of anxieties about zoonosis and, as we shall see, about human nature that have been expressed in relation to the practice of animal to human organ donation. The difference can be understood partly in terms of the biological nature of the animal body part that is being transplanted. Pig valves, for example, are less likely to transmit infection to humans and are less likely to be rejected by the human body. The valves are cartilaginous and can be freeze dried. Unlike organs such as hearts, valves do not have to be transplanted 'live', i.e. immediately following removal from the animal (R. Lentil, personal communication, 31 October, 2005; M. Short, personal communication, 30 October, 2005). As devices that open, close or regulate flow, heart valves are tissues through which the life-blood *passes*, but they do not carry the same symbolic weight as the heart itself that is responsible for pumping blood around the body.

The last couple of decades have seen pig's skin used to help burn victims without generating fears about zoonosis. Medical procedures are such that skin is less likely to carry and communicate infection and less likely to provoke immune rejection. It might also be instructive to think about the symbolism of skin. Before the nineteenth century, the surface of the body, the skin, was invested with a meaning very different to modern meanings, and this meaning was connected to a particular way of thinking about the body. Bakhtin (1984) contrasts the 'grotesque' conception of the body found in medieval European popular culture with modern conceptions of the body. The 'grotesque' body intermingled with the world. Protruding body parts such as the stomach or nose were seen as projecting into the world, while the inside of the body moved outwards, also mingling with the world. The body was 'open' and the skin was understood as a porous layer with a multitude of possible openings: eyes, ears, nose, mouth, breasts, anus, urinary passage and vulva. Relating this conception of the body to the skin, Benthien observes that the skin was fragile, and it was a boundary, but it was not perceived as demarcating the body *against* the world. The 'inside' revealed itself on the surface of the body and the surface was 'a place of permeability and mysterious metamorphosis' (Benthien 2002: 39). Links between the body as microcosm in relationship to the macro surrounding it were deeply embedded in culture. The relationship between the 'inside' and 'outside' was seen in terms of a kind of living exchange. The skin stood metonymically for the whole human being and the word 'skin' was at times used instead of 'person' (Benthien 2002: 23) so that the skin in one form or another was thought of as representing the self, characterized as a 'surface entity'.

Although there clearly are differences in terms of lived experience and competing ideologies and discourses, Bakhtin views the modern conception of the body as being quite different to the popular medieval conception. He describes the bourgeois body as 'an entirely finished, completed, strictly limited body, which is shown from the outside as something individual. That which protrudes, bulges, sprouts or branches off ... is eliminated, hidden or moderated. All orifices of the body are closed' (1984: 319–20). The bourgeois body is strictly demarcated, with a smooth impenetrable exterior. It is a body that is 'closed' to the world, totally individual and non-merging. Whereas popular medieval conceptions connected the body inextricably to nature, the modern body became an individual possession with a façade of opaque impenetrability.

As the body was delineated in this way, in the twentieth century skin became the central metaphor of separateness, a boundary and contact surface. Benthien sees the 'change of skin within the history of mentalities as a move from a porous, tissue like membrane to an impenetrable wall of separation' (2002: 14). The skin became simultaneously the 'other' of self; an enclosure of self, a prison or mask of self. One level of meaning for the skin in some expressions found within European languages is that of concealment and deceit. What is authentic is thought to lie beneath the skin, hidden inside the body. Here skin is conceived as something other than the self, as something foreign and external to it. Acting as impenetrable armour, the skin becomes a boundary or barrier against the world with an individuated self-contained inner space of the body. The symbolic smoothing of the body and hardening of its external boundaries demarcated the individual body with a final boundary of the skin.

Pigs and privatized and pluralized psyches

This historical shift in the conceptualization of the body, moving from 'open' to 'closed', together with the shift in the symbolic nature of the skin, moving from permeability and porosity to boundary and barrier occurred at the same time as an increased delineation of the privatized psyche. The eighteenth and nineteenth centuries marked the emergence of the modern 'self', experienced on the inside and separate from the outside. The authentic character of a person, their core and essence, their real self, was now located within the inner space and inner world of the individual person.

Allusions to this kind of understanding and experience of the self have been expressed by human organ recipients who report changes in their subjective sense of who they are as a consequence of organ transplantation (Lock 1995; Sharpe 1995). However, this experience also alludes to a more fluid or 'liquid' (Bauman 2000) sense of self, a fluidity and liquidity perhaps expressed in the immune system, which, while '... maintaining individual bodily coherence ... is everywhere and nowhere ... [in] ... a network-body of truly amazing complexity and specificity ...' (Haraway 1991: 218). The 'postmodern' self, more fragmented in terms of symbolic consistency and narrative texture, is characterized by ambiguities, ambivalence, discontinuity, dread, flux, multiplicity and turmoil. The 'self' may be recognized as a composite of contending discourses, practices, representations, images and fantasies (Elliott 2001).

I would argue that both of these senses of self, the 'modern' and the 'postmodern' are embedded in our fears of xenozoonosis. Given the symbolic significance of human organs for self-identity, part of the concern about transplanting animal organs into humans might be to do with perceptions that this challenges boundaries that have been drawn between ourselves and other species in modern society. We may fear that we are in danger of making 'other' animals of ourselves. While not wanting to underestimate or minimize the danger that xenozoonosis may pose, I would also suggest that we might view anxieties about xenozoonosis as a reflection of our own 'shadow', a 'shadow' that we project onto other animals.

The pig, currently the preferred source of organs for xenotransplantation, has, as Caspari (2003) outlines, long been the object of contradictory or ambivalent human projections. In its negative aspect it is the archetype and prime metaphor of greed, indulgence and behaviour deemed to be socially unacceptable. Negative associations of the pig have been highlighted in myth. In Egyptian mythology, for example, the black pig was considered

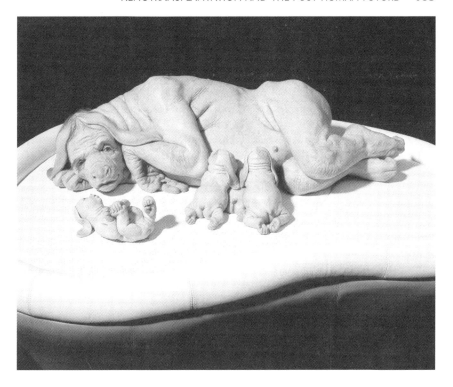

Figure 9.1 'The Young Family'

Source: Patricia Piccinini. Reprinted with kind permission.

unclean and forbidden as food. In ancient Chinese culture, the pig re-presented raw untamed nature, dirty and avaricious. In the *I Ching*, the Chinese *Book of Changes*, the pig symbolizes the 'Abysmal', a fall, danger or a great chasm. In both Judaism and Islam the pig is regarded as unclean. In Christianity the pig has been associated with the Devil, symbolizing sensuality and gluttony. The pig may remind us of ourselves in different ways. Today, part of their preferred status as organ 'donors' is to do with their anatomical and physiological similarity to humans. In the Middle Ages, dead pigs were used for medical instruction, the internal organs being layed out similarly to those of humans. As Caspari points out, the pig can also seem like a grotesque parody of human self-indulgence with its pink and usually hairless, rotund, fleshy body, and greedy physical and sexual appetites (Caspari 2003). Our fears of xenozoonosis may warn us of the dangers of our own 'piggishness'.

Other oracles, ourselves and Odysseus

In 1996 the Nuffield Council on Bioethics established an Advisory Group to assess the risks to the public of cross-species, that is, animal to human, infection. The Advisory Group came to the conclusion that clinical trials of xenotransplantation were not appropriate because of insufficient information about the immune response of humans and the physiological behaviour of xenografts. Uppermost in their deliberations was the risk of cross-species infection. Nuffield advised that the risks of cross-species infection were such that trials of animal to human xenotransplantation would be unethical. Nonetheless, Nuffield also recommended that non-primate species should be the source of organs for xenotransplantation. In both of these re-commendations human interest was prioritized over the interests of other animals. The recommendation to halt clinical trials of xenotransplantation was clearly made in the interests of humans, and the recommendation con-cerning non-primate species was based upon the speciest interest of primates. The privileging of the human species is clearly evident in the principles that were used to guide Nuffield's position with respect to xenotransplantation. The use of animals for medical purposes was seen as 'an undesirable but unavoidable necessity' and 'in the absence of any scientifically and morally acceptable alternative, some use of animals . . . can be justified as necessary to safeguard and improve the health and alleviate the suffering of human beings' (Nuffield Council on Bioethics 1996: 1).

From an anthropocentric and speciest point of view there may seem to be little difference between breeding non-human animals for food and breeding non-human animals for the purposes of organ transplantation. Indeed, ani-mal ethicist Peter Singer suggests that, 'If society believed it's OK to raise pigs in factories in order to give people bacon for their breakfast, then they will think it's even more justifiable to do it to give people kidneys' (O'Neill 2006: 221). Research certainly indicates a willingness to accept animal organs for transplantation. A study by Ward (1997), for example, of 858 patients found that 87 per cent were willing to accept a pig's kidney. Similarly the National Kidney Federation (1995, cited in Long *et al.* 2002) in the USA found that transplant recipients were more likely to accept a xenograft if they needed another transplant and a human organ was unavailable.

However, in a recent study of the attitudes of 100 patients and their caregivers to xenotransplantation involving hearts and lungs (Long *et al.* 2002), patients indicated that they would find it more difficult to accept an organ from an animal. One patient expressed the view that it is not acceptable to mix human and animal organs. When asked if they would be willing to accept an animal organ, most patients and caregivers did not respond. Long *et al.* suggest 'That . . . our population did not comment when asked if they would accept a xenograft may support the view that the heart is seen differently from other organs and that the issue of having a pig's heart is therefore more difficult to contemplate' (Long *et al.* 2002: 284). I would suggest that this difficulty might be connected to the archetypal significance of the heart. Visioned in the West as the seat of the soul or the self, the heart also carries a certain numinous significance. Consequently we may intuit the replacement of a human heart with, say, the heart of a pig, as a sacrilegious act.

Xenotransplantation involving major organs such as hearts also opens up the 'heart' of another matter, namely vivisection. Research among potential xenotransplantation recipients on the use of animals for human benefit indicates agreement with animal experimentation and killing animals for human benefit (Long *et al.* 2002). In research by Mohacsi *et al.* (1995, 1997), out of a sample of 113 patients, 48 per cent thought that it was acceptable to breed animals to provide organs for transplantation. However, in the study by Ward (1997), misgivings about breeding animals solely for organ replacement was the most reported concern. In the study by Long *et al.* the main problem about xenotransplantation identified by patients and caregivers was the ethics and morality of killing animals for transplantation into humans. As one patient said, 'Just because we can does not mean that we should' (Long *et al.* 2002: 287).

Vivisection for medical research is usually hidden in the liminal space of the laboratory. In that space, through the alchemy of science, animal mortality and morbidity is transformed into elixirs of life, from which any traces of the sacrificial animals are, so it is believed, exorcised. Just as cooking metamorphoses meat into an artefact of culinary culture (Levi-Strauss 1970), the application of science and medicine metamorphoses animal morbidity and inanimate, dead, animal bodies into substances to sustain human life. However, fears about xenozoonosis and concerns about using animals as organ donors may, in part, be shaped by an intuition that this alchemical transformation might not be so successfully effected by xenotransplantation, particularly where it involves major organs such as hearts. Our anxieties and concerns might express a subliminal unease about the possibility that the spirits of dead animal ancestors and kin will return to haunt us. The image of a human being with a pig's heart '*in situ*' may invoke memories of monstrous metamorphosis from our mythological past. Rather than activating the positive ancient mythological porcine projections of fertility and fecundity, we may be haunted by the possibility of a fate similar to that of Odysseus' men: men who were turned into pigs by the sorceress Circe after gorging themselves at a feast. Science and technology may deliver us a lot closer to the corporeal expression of archetypes of animality than the myths of metamorphoses that populate our collective unconscious, sending us back down the evolutionary chain, and alchemizing the archaic and ultra-modern into mercurial forms of our own embodied animality.

Conclusion

The figure of the animal-human hybrid is an ancient one. The archetypal amalgam of man and beast is steeped in mythological and religious belief. It is also reflected in scientific practice, as the history of xenotransplantation demonstrates. To date, animal to human xenografts of major organs have not worked, but this does not seem to obviate human imaginings about the possibility of a post-human future that technologies such as xenotransplantation may conjure up. In this respect our imagination might be ignited and persuaded by the timelessness of some of the messages embedded in ancient myth, drawing on them to think about practices such as xenotransplantation. In both contemporary times and in any post-human future yet to come, these ancient myths could be read as a timeless message of hope for humans and other species.

Acknowledgement

Thanks to Stuart Hubbard for listening to my ideas and providing invaluable technical support.

References

Bakhtin, M. (1984) *Rabelais and His World*. Bloomington, IN: Indiana University Press.
Bauman, Z. (2000) *Liquid Modernity*. Cambridge: Polity Press.
Benthien, C. (2002) *Skin on the Cultural Border Between Self and the World*. New York: Columbia State University Press.
Caspari, E. (2003) *Animal Life in Nature, Myth and Dreams*. Wilmette, IL: Chiron.
Champsaur, F. (1929) *Nora, la guenon devenue femme* (*Nora, the Female Ape Who Became a Woman*). Paris: Ferenczi et fils.
Corrigan, P. and Sayer, D. (1985) *The Great Arch*. Oxford: Basil Blackwell.
Dartigues, L. (1925) *La Greffe de revitalisation humaine* (*Graft for Human Revitalization*). Paris: Gaston Doin editeur.
Deschamps, J.Y., Roux, F.A., Sai, P. and Gouin, E. (2005) History of xenotransplantation, *Xenotransplantation*, 12(2): 91–109.
Douglas, M. (1978) *Purity and Danger: An Analysis of Concepts of Pollution and Taboo*. London: Routledge & Kegan Paul.
Elliott, A. (2001) *Concepts of the Self*. Cambridge: Polity Press.
Farr, A.D. (1980) The first human blood transfusion, *Medical History*, 24(2): 143–62.
Germond, P. (2001) *An Egyptian Bestiary*. London: Thames & Hudson.

Guirand, F. (1970) Greek mythology, in R. Graves *New Larousse Encyclopedia of Mythology*. London: Hamlyn.

Hancock, G. (2005) *Supernatural*. London: Random House.

Haraway, D. (1989) *Primate Visions: Gender, Race and Nature in the World of Modern Science*. London: Routledge.

Haraway, D. (1991) *Simians, Cyborgs, and Women: The Reinvention of Nature*. London: Free Association Books.

Jones, O. (2000) (Un)ethical geographies of human-non-human relations: encounters, collectives and spaces, in C. Philo and C. Wilbert (eds) *Animal Spaces, Beastly Places: New Geographies of Human-Animal Relations*. London: Routledge.

Kafka, F. (1961) *The Metamorphosis and Other Stories*. Harmondsworth: Penguin.

Keys, T.E. (1973) Dr Paul Bert (1833–1886), *Anesthesia & Analgesia*, 52: 437–8.

Kuss, R. and Bourget, P. (1992) *Une histoire illustree de la greffe d'organes. La grande adventure du siecle. (An Illustrated History of Organ Transplantation: The Great Adventure of the Century)*. Rueil-Malmaison, France: Laboratoires Sandoz.

Levi-Strauss, C. (1970) *The Raw and the Cooked*. London: Cape.

Lewis, C.S. (1993) *The Lion, the Witch and the Wardrobe*. London: Lions.

Lock, M. (1995) Transcending mortality: organ transplants and the practice of contradictions, *Medical Anthropology Quarterly*, 9(3): 390–3.

Long, T., Wray, J., Myers, L. and Banner, N. (2002) Attitudes of potential candidates for heart and heart-lung transplantation to xenotransplantation, *Progress in Transplantation*, 12(4): 280–8.

Mac Cana, P. (1984) *Celtic Mythology*. Middlesex: Hamlyn.

Mekdeci, B. (1997) *Nostradamus: The Great Visionary*. http://aries.phys.yorku.ca/~mmdr/1800/nostradamus.html (accessed 31 July 2006).

Mohacsi, P.J., Blumer, C.E., Quine, S. and Thompson, J. (1995) Aversion to xenotransplantation, *Nature*, 378: 434.

Mohacsi, P.J., Thompson, J.F., Nicholson, J.K. and Tiller, D.J. (1997) Patients' attitudes to xenotransplantation, *The Lancet*, 349: 1031.

Murray, M. (1995) *The Law of the Father?* London: Routledege.

Neuhof, H. (1923) *The Transplantation of Tissues*. New York: Appleton.

Nuffield Council on Bioethics (1996) *Animal-to-Human Transplants: the Ethics of Xenotransplantation*. London: Nuffield Council on Bioethics.

O'Neill, R.D. (2006) Xenotransplantation: the solution to the shortage of human organs for transplantation? *Mortality*, 11(2): 211–31.

Philo, C. and Wilbert, C. (2000) *Animal Spaces, Beastly Places: New Geographies of Human-Animal Relations*. London: Routledge.

Piccinini, P. (2006) *In Another Life*. Wellington: City Gallery.

Said, E. (1978) *Orientalism*. London: Routledge & Kegan Paul.

Salisbury, J.E. (1994) *The Beast Within: Animals in the Middle Ages*. London: Routledge.

Sharpe, L.A. (1995) Organ transplantation as a transformative experience: an-thropological insights into the restructuring of the self, *Medical Anthropological Quarterly*, 9(3): 357–89.

Shildrick, M. (2002) *Embodying the Monster: Encounters with the Vulnerable Self*. London: Sage.

Somerville, M. (2000) *The Ethical Canary: Science, Society and the Human Spirit*. Middlesex: Penguin.

Tolkien, J.R.R. (1995) *The Lord of The Rings*. London: HarperCollins.

Voronoff, S. (1924) *Quarante-trois greffes du singe a l'homme (Forty-three ape-to-man transplantations)*. Paris: Gaston Doin editeur.

Ward, E. (1997) Attitudes to xenotransplantation, *The Lancet*, 349: 1775.

Wolfe, C. (2003) *Animal Rites, American Culture, the Discourse of Species and Post-humanist Theory*. Chicago: University of Chicago Press.

10 Closing thoughts and the future

Magi Sque and Sheila Payne

Introduction

The preceding chapters have discussed current issues in organ donation and transplantation and provided a detailed evidence base to support good practice for health professionals and others working in this field. Richardson set the context for the book by providing a historical backdrop to organ donation and transplantation. The early chapters contributed theoretical insights that highlighted the tensions that may exist for potential donor families between giving 'the gift of life' or making a 'sacrifice', bereavement and the dissonant loss associated with organ donation. From the chapters that follow a picture emerges of organ and tissue donation and transplantation as a rapidly developing health care innovation at the cutting edge of bio-technological development and the human needs and controversies inherent in these developments.

This chapter will discuss the implications of further advances in new technologies to the development of organ donation and transplantation. It will provide an understanding of psychological and social issues that under-pin these important health interventions. It will seek to highlight some of the ongoing and potential debates and areas of research, which individuals interested in and working in this developing health field should be aware of so that appropriate policies and health systems can be developed to protect and support families and individuals faced with choices about organ and tissue donation.

The future of organ and tissue replacement

Human organ transplantation was undoubtedly one of the outstanding medico-surgical advances of the twentieth century offering individuals, facing certain death from end stage organ failure, a second chance of life. A victim of its own success means that the worldwide demand for viable organs has grown exponentially and donation rates have not kept pace with demand, leading to an increasing number of potentially preventable deaths. Niklason and Langer (2001) also noted that an additional burden of need for available organs is due in part to the progressive ageing population in many countries around the world, with the concurrent age-related degeneration of organs. They propose that expansion of the donor pool, even with extended criteria to older donors, is unlikely.

No discussion designed to capture the most important current issues concerning organ donation and transplantation would be complete without the consideration of living donation where organs such as livers or kidneys are donated by a living person to save the life of another. Without this avenue to transplantation an increasing number of individuals would face certain death, as living donation now forms an important source of organs. Living donation also remains preferable in some countries such as Japan (Lock 2002) and Mexico (Crowley-Matoka and Lock 2006), due to cultural and legal frameworks that make donation from cadaveric organs problematic. However, as Franklin and Crombie (Chapter 8) have discussed, living donation still poses significant challenges and risks to family relationships and the donor, and is therefore likely to remain a limited contribution, confined to specialist centres.

So there can be no doubt that transplantation of human organs or tissue from the living or the dead will remain an important therapy for the foreseeable future and the reason that the promotion of organ donation has become the concern of many health systems across the globe. A number of recent consultations also point to the importance of improving and trying to find pragmatic solutions to the donor shortage. The World Health Organization (WHO) is currently consulting to update its *Guiding Principles on Transplantation*; the European Union (EU) has launched a public consultation to identify the main problems encountered in organ donation and transplantation and to determine the extent to which measures should be taken at EU level to help to solve these problems; and the Economic and Social Research Council (ESRC), the UK's leading research and training agency, has recently funded a University of Manchester School of Law seminar series, for two years: 'ESRC Seminar Series: Transplantation and the Organ Deficit in the UK: Pragmatic Solutions to Ethical Controversy', to debate and find possible solutions to the UK donor shortage.

Clearly with no present resolution to the constraints of the donor pool, methods to make the best use of organs that do become available and new avenues for development are being sought. Improved surgical techniques, use of immunosuppressive agents, organ preservation, advances in molecular immunology, tissue engineering and stem cell biology are thought to be among the developments that will offer a bright future to treating organ failure (Niklason and Langer 2001). Enhanced understanding of the immune tolerance of transplanted tissues, further insight into cellular differentiation, tissue development and advances in biomaterials may lead to the creation of new types of implantable materials. The contribution of these new techniques to improving transplantation outcomes, reducing the number of re-transplants, should consequently assist in the reduction of transplant waiting lists (Niklason and Langer 2001).

Research on cellular transplants continues apace, for instance pancreatic islets cells can be transplanted into the liver where they produce insulin to control diabetes, one of the leading causes of renal failure (UK Transplant 2005). Work is also developing the use of limbal epithelial cells transplantation (Tsai *et al.* 2000). Small numbers of cells can be removed from a healthy eye, grown in the laboratory, and then used to treat a damaged eye, instead of corneal replacement from another person (UK Transplant 2005).

Advances in mechanical artificial organs such as replacement heart pumps and the use of animal livers have improved the treatment of organ failure, but they are unable to perform all of the functions of a single organ; therefore they can still only act as brief respite bridges to human transplantation.

In the UK the Human Tissue Act (2004) that overhauled previous laws with regard to the use of human organs. It has opened the way for the cannulation and mechanical restoration of the heartbeat, following the dead donor rule criteria, of dead bodies to assist the non-heartbeating organ donation programme. However, the USA and UK still trail behind Spain in the use of donors that become available through uncontrolled non-heartbeating donation (Matesanz and Miranda 2002). With a controlled non-heartbeating programme only tentatively established, uncontrolled non-hearting donation raises a completely new arena for education of health professionals and the public. Both health professionals' and the public's perception and acceptance warrant investigation from a number of perspectives.

The use of animal organs (xenotranplantation) is still not clinically available and the social and ethical issues with which society must grapple and as Murray debates in Chapter 10 threaten our very sense of what is means to be human. How far will we accept the mixing and alteration of the human and animal gene pool? Will human chimeras developed from a variety of animals become the norm and even desirable? Transplantation medicine as an innovation is still in its infancy but the rapid progression of the technology leaves us in no doubt that the future possibilities cannot yet even be imagined.

There is also a new class of body parts that have become available for transplantation, which are likely to open floodgates of demand and raise novel questions about the sanctity of the living and dead body and what may be reasonable to remove and use. For instance, composite tissue transplants of hands and forearms have been a reality in certain specialist transplant centres since 1999. The first face transplant using skin from another person, carried out in France by a team led by Bernard Devauchelle and Jean Michel Dubernard on the 27 November 2005 (Spurgeon 2005; Devauchelle *et al.* 2006), was not without controversy. As recently as 2003 surgeons in England had called for a moratorium on face transplants (Clark 2005), as it was widely recognized that face transplantation is more than a technical achievement. Concerns relating to the psychological impact on donor families and recipients, lifelong immunosuppression and the consequence of technical failure have so far prevented ethical approval of the procedure in some countries, although the microsurgical skills and anatomical knowledge is well established and surgeons are fully able to perform such transplants. Doctors working in the field say many could benefit from the procedure (Clark 2005), including 10,000 burns victims in the UK alone (www. BBC news/health, 30 November 2005). Clark has pointed out that while surgeons wanting to do face transplants argue 'how they should proceed' other stakeholders are asking 'should they proceed?'.

Richardson has shown clearly in her chapter that where there is demand, market forces both legal and illegal are likely to intervene. So it is that human organ and tissue transplantation has expanded to embrace an immense enterprise around the world for both life-saving and life-enhancing purposes via both the legal and illegal brokerage of body parts (Scheper-Hughes 2000; Youngner *et al.* 2004; Cheney 2006). The scale of world trade in human body parts and tissues that are easily transported across borders and countries has become a concern to regulators and legislators and could be detrimental to the whole transplantation programme.[1] Not only does this raise the sceptre of need for integrated control systems between countries (a recent concern of the WHO)[2] but it also touches on our perceptions of humanity and if body parts should be ascribed a commercial value.

The tissue bank trade is a lucrative business, with body parts, subject to family consent and medical checks, now an integral part of routine operations, from heart surgery to dental implants. More than 19,000 square feet of skin were distributed in 2003 from transplant accredited tissue banks, according to the American Association of Tissue Banks, up from 7700 square feet in 1999. Approximately 3300 heart valves were distributed in 2003, up from 1300 in 1999 (Armour 2006). Tumours and excess tissue that were once incinerated as waste can now be probed for DNA markers, to help doctors understand disease.

Campbell (2006) writes that tissue banking in the USA is in crisis with the introduction of for-profit companies in the distribution and marketing of tissue. His belief is that the crossing over of this humanitarian effort into the commercial arena will have lasting and adverse effects on the efforts of all transplant organizations by establishing a negative image of the transplant community in the public's eye. While many people in the industry may, themselves, find it repugnant to refer to human tissue as a 'commodity', the language and ingrained patterns of discourse are those of objectification, turning human tissue into a 'product' or 'medical device' that will be profitable goods for company shareholders.

The questions that arise from this market are about the process of the 'devaluing' of the human body that in life represented a unique individual. In most countries priceless human body parts and tissues are procured through a donation, most likely facilitated by a grieving family. These body parts or tissues through processing acquire a market value that allows them to be bought or sold as property. At what point in this process is the line crossed from human body parts or tissue to 'raw material' and 'product'? How well informed are the public about such practices that they are truly able to give informed consent at donation? Kent and Wells *et al.* (Chapters 6, 7) alerted us to the limited knowledge that health professionals, themselves, have about these processes. Should we accept the commodification of the dead body in the light of what history teaches us, such as the dangers that lay at the heart of the Burke and Hare murders?

While organ transplantation is well regulated in most countries worldwide, by comparison tissue transplantation is not. Body parts are valuable enough that theft occurs. Although it is illegal to buy and sell tissue, those involved in tissue theft manage this by exploiting loopholes that allow 'modern-day body snatchers' to provide bones, tendons and body parts to tissue banks, research facilities and other buyers charging an unspecified processing fee for handling, storing and transporting human tissue (Cheney 2006). This commercial trade in organs, tissues and body parts refocuses our thinking on the disreputable history of bodies snatched from graveyards or people murdered to supply anatomy schools for use in medical training (Richardson 2001). Just like the eighteenth-century resurrectionists, to modern-day entrepreneurs bodies and tissue can be a boon in education. Fresh corpses, for instance, are preferred to 'rubbery' embalmed bodies to teach doctors laparoscopic surgery. The use of stolen body parts is a risky business as implanted into humans they can potentially expose recipients to HIV, hepatitis and syphilis and other diseases as death certificates and other relevant documents are often falsified to match donor criteria.

Recently the high profile case concerning the well-known British-American broadcaster, Alistair Cooke, who died in America, was reported in *The Sunday Times* on 12 March 2006 (Cooke Kittredge 2006). His body became the subject of a police investigation into the illegal sale of 1077 bodies by several funeral homes, when it was discovered that his legs had been cut off and sold. The body parts from this investigation were traded as far afield as the UK, Ireland and other European countries. Investigators found that Cooke's age had been changed to a decade younger from 95 to 85 and his cause of death was changed from lung cancer that had metastasized to his bones to a heart attack, both to seemingly fit donor criteria. A consent form was also falsified. The case turned the spotlight onto a secret global industry. In 2006 Senator Charles Schumer called for regulatory oversight after another case came to light where a tissue service was found to have solicited funeral homes to illegally provide body parts (Armour 2006).

Issues for a new age of transplantation

The role of the family in consent

Relatives of potential deceased donors have been and will remain a critical link in maintaining organ supply, as organ donation is normally discussed with them and their support for, agreement or lack of an objection sought, before donation takes place. However, legislation enacted in the UK through the Human Tissue Act (2004) now gives precedence to the wishes of the deceased in any donation decision and families can be advised that they have no right to veto those wishes. We wait to see how this 'rolls out' in practice, and whether health professionals in the UK will be prepared to override the wishes of a bereaved family. Recent research has shown that in 9 cases out of 23, families chose not to donate organs or tissue, although they were aware that in life the deceased had wished to be an organ donor (Sque *et al.* 2006). This was a surprising finding in a small study. If this finding was extrapolated to all families with whom donation is discussed it could help account for many negative decisions that impact the availability of organs.

A recently published exploratory study (Dodd-McCue *et al.* 2006) tracked the results of legislative changes in the state of Virginia, USA, over five years. These changes reinforced the rights of the deceased by mandating that their wish in life to be a donor should be strictly honoured. The research showed that donors' families, who responded to the self-complete survey (162 of 569 families, 27 per cent), were not negatively affected by the strict enforcement of a donor's wishes. In fact these families perceived the situation as less stressful when they were aware and informed of their relative's wishes to be an organ donor rather than being requested to make the donation. While these results must be viewed with caution as 70 per cent of all donor families failed to respond and it is unclear whether those families who did respond differ from those who did not, the response rate nevertheless compares favourably with other self-completion mail surveys.

Virginia legislation changes the emphasis in the donation discussion with families from one of 'request' to 'informing'. Dodd-McCue *et al.* (2006) suggested that US organ procurement organizations and donor professionals, even though supported by legislation, remain reluctant to change their donation discussion practices, fearing legal or other negative repercussions from next of kin. However, other recent work in the USA where the wishes of the deceased have been given precedent and the wishes of the family have been set aside, has shown that families are grateful when they have had time to think about their decision and are pleased that the wishes of their deceased relative were upheld, at a time when they were too overcome with grief to respond appropriately (Personal communication with Gunderson 2005). Other countries like Canada have argued in favour of such a policy for many years (Kluge 1997). The policy is already available within Canadian law but in practice the wishes of the bereaved family are always carried out. While the above findings suggest that upholding the deceased's wishes can lead to positive results for donor families, as well as transplant recipients, there is room for a more rigorous evidence base to support this practice and consequently instil confidence in the health professionals' donation discussions with families.

The family's role in decision-making

Families may be asked to make new decisions about donation in the future with regard to the use of composite tissue. These decisions, as yet few, are set to become more frequent. The increasing longevity of allografts and the return of functionality of hands, and hands with forearms following transplantation, and the first successful face transplant, mean that there will be the potential for this field of transplantation to expand. Some would argue however that these allografts, because only a few have been performed, still occupy the realm of research and cannot yet be regarded as therapy (Dickenson and Widdershoven 2001).

Decisions made by families about composite tissue remain uninvestigated but could be expected to be particularly difficult. Both the hand and the face occupy privileged positions as vehicles for the expression of personal identity and intimacy. Issues these decisions may pose for bereaved families are about whether they are contributing to research or therapy. A research focus may impinge on the 'sacrifice' they are prepared to make. Carving up the body is already perceived by bereaved families as a form of mutilation, which may only be acceptable because it saves somebody's life (Sque *et al.* 2005, 2006). Unlike organ transplants limb allografts are not lifesaving, although face transplants may be.

There is also the issue of seeing the face of the deceased on another person. While these transplants are expected to create a hybrid face between that of the donor and the recipient, the amount of publicity and the donation discussion with the family will mean that the anonymity of the recipient and donor will be difficult to ensure. The aesthetic presentation of the corpse could also prove problematic. Even with the substitution of prostheses the visible mutilation of the corpse and the consequent perceived spoiled identity and integrity of the person the corpse represents creates an unnaturalness of a body without a face or hands. It may also be unsettling to think that the face or hand with which one was once intimate may now respectively be stroked by or stroke another body (Dickenson and Widdershoven 2001).

Altman writes in the *New York Times* (26 January 2006) all that seems to be 'publicly' known about the family who donated the first hand for transplant in the USA, to a man who lost his hand in a fireworks accident: 'Elizabeth Reed, the Regional Director for Kentucky Organ Affiliates, the procurement agency stated 'It was a very caring family who wanted to help'. Undoubtedly limb and face transplants are not ethically straightforward. They pose deep dilemmas for families about autonomy, identity and bodily integrity and will require a great deal of effort from all involved (Dickenson and Widdershoven 2001). On a more general level the impact on society of the possibilities of new appearance-enhancing procedures should not be underestimated (Rumsey 2004). For instance, will 'changing faces' become accepted routine practice for therapeutic and cosmetic pursuits or will such practice remain in the realms of fiction and entertainment?

What tissue donation and its use means to families

With the possibility of a new era of tissue transplantation it is important to know what tissue donation and its use means to families. Although there have been many studies that have examined the experiences of families of organ donors, there is still little information in regard to families of tissue donors. Beard *et al.* (2002) were unable to identify any study in which the majority of participants were tissue-only donors. Despite this lack of focused research into the experiences and needs of tissue donor families, Haire and Hinchliff (1996) claimed that the needs of these families were the same as for organ donor families in terms of the need for a sensitive discussion about donation, information-giving and follow-up bereavement support. However, none of these studies had elicited the importance of the donation of even small pieces of tissue to the family.

In 1999, UK post-mortem procedures were placed under a spotlight. During an investigation into the care of children receiving complex cardiac surgery at the Bristol Royal Infirmary (Department of Health 2001), it was disclosed that organs and tissues had been retained without the knowledge and explicit consent of the next of kin. This disclosure triggered inquiries into the practice of other NHS Hospital Trusts and coroners' services. It was found that hearts, brains and other organs had been routinely removed at post-mortem and stored for the purposes of further investigations, research and teaching (Redfern 2001; Retained Organs Commission 2002a, 2002b). In 2001 a nationwide census revealed that 105,000 organs, body parts or pre-term babies were held by pathology services (Ramsay 2001). These revelations sparked widespread concern among families, with some 30,000 contacting the hospitals in which their babies, children or relative had died, to ask if their organs had been retained (Retained Organs Commission 2002c).

What was enlightening about these phenomena was the difference in parents' attitudes to small pieces of tissue that had been retained from their children and that of some health professionals. To parents even the smallest piece of retained tissue remained part of their child or pre-term baby and not objects of laboratory information, i.e. blocks and slides or foetuses. Parents wanted to be involved in the use and future disposal of these parts of their children (Sque *et al.* 2004). Parents reported that the sanctity of organs was diminished by the actions of health care professionals as well as the terminology used to discuss babies' or children's retained organs. Parents explained that the use of terms such as 'body parts' and 'trimmings' devalued the person that was their baby or child.

Parents' attitudes may provide clues to the respect families may feel should be paid to even the smallest cell or tissue donated by their deceased relative. So the quality of tissue donation is not only an ethical issue for the recipient but for the donor and the donor family as well. If tissue is taken from a dead donor then because of the perceived mutilation and the 'preciousness' of the donated tissue the family have a right to expect the very best use of that tissue to be made. The reconstruction process and aesthetic presentation of the body should also consider the feelings of the bereaved family.

Organ and tissue donation depends to a large extent on the wish of a donor in life or the generosity of a bereaved family at a time during which they could be expected to be engulfed by great sadness and sorrow. Bereaved families with whom it is appropriate to discuss tissue donation should therefore expect to only be approached by individuals who are educated to work with the bereaved; professionals who are confident in this role and *comfortable* discussing donation with families, not only *trained* to do so. Assessment of the family's information needs, the family dynamics and recognition of the main decision-maker is crucial to fulfil the family's needs, evaluate their ability to process and use information and ensure the discussion about donation is timely and sensitive. The 'requestor' needs to be available to the family during their decision-making to support them, answer their questions and provide the family with a contact where they can *easily* access further information should they have the need. 'Requestors' therefore need to be skilled at enabling family members to talk openly about issues and make choices with the recognition that the circumstances of loss and bereavement are culturally challenging, especially the post-mortem procedures on the body. Follow-up support for the family and their information needs should be negotiated. Families should expect that the contribution of their deceased relative is recognized, valued and not forgotten.

The last word

The process of organ donation and transplantation is complex and demanding for all involved because human bodies and organs have value to the individual, the family, the potential recipient, research and society. It also calls into question some of our taken for grantedness about the body and challenges us to think about such issues. For instance, we both 'are' and 'have' a body; experienced through living in a body that defines our identity. These challenges translate into the respect we hold for the preferences of the donor and their family, the promotion of a sense of societal generosity and improving the quality of life for those who could benefit from transplantation.

Technological advances have raised many philosophical, moral, psychological and social concerns for society at large, and for the people directly affected through the transplantation process. Fundamental issues such as the definition of life and death, the market value of human tissue, the rationing of health care resources, the ethics of donor recruitment and care and the use of animals for transplantation have all been widely debated. Less attention has been focused on the psychological and social effects of the donation and transplantation process on bereaved families, recipients and involved health professionals. These sensitive research fields warrant further investigation, so that appropriate policies can be adopted, particularly with regard to the many controversial and emerging biomedical techniques, as they become available.

This book has sought to provide an evidence base and to provoke thought about some of the important issues that concern organ donation and transplantation in today's world and to highlight more clearly new avenues for research; research that is needed to further understand the roles of individuals in the donation-transplantation process and how they are affected by it.

Challenges for the future will be about trying to find ways to narrow the gap between organ demand and supply and the control of global organ and tissue markets that prey upon vulnerable communities, including the dead. Research is therefore also needed to further inform and understand the complexities of the organization of this medico-surgical field to provide safeguards for the vulnerable individuals who may be caught up in the organ transplant process and their probable use as organ sources, as this field inevitably develops throughout the twenty-first century.

Note

1   Readers wishing to engage in a detailed analysis of this issue are advised to read Youngner, S.J., Anderson, M.W. and Schapiro, R. (eds) (2004)

Transplanting Human Tissue: Ethics, Policy and Practice. Oxford: Oxford University Press.

2 WHO called for evidence of illegal trade in organs at the ESOT Conference in Geneva, October, 2005. WHO sponsored a symposium to discuss international policy for regulation of tissue donation, storage and use in Zurich, July, 2006.

References

Armour, S. (2006) Illegal trade in bodies shakes loved ones, *USA Today.* www.usatoday.com/money/2006–04–26-body-parts-cover-usat_x.htm (accessed 6 June 2006).

Beard, J., Ireland, L., Davis, N. and Barr, J. (2002) Tissue donation: what it means to families, *Progress in Transplantation*, 12(1): 42–8.

Campbell, C. S. (2006) The gift and the market: cultural symbolic perspectives, in S. J. Youngner, M.W. Anderson and R. Schapiro (eds) *Transplanting Human Tissue: Ethics, Policy and Practice.* Oxford: Oxford University Press.

Cheney, A. (2006) *Body Brokers: Inside America's Underground Trade in Human Remains.* New York: Broadway.

Clark, P.A. (2005) Face transplantation: Part II – an ethical perspective, *Medical Science Monitor*, 11: 2, RA41–7.

Cooke Kittredge, S. (2006) Dad and the bodysnatchers, News Review, The *Sunday Times*, 4.3, 12 March.

Crowley-Matoka, M. and Lock, M. (2006) Organ transplantation in a globalised world, *Mortality*, 11(2): 166–81.

Department of Health (2001) *The Report of the Bristol Royal Infirmary Inquiry.* London: DoH.

Devauchelle, B., Badet, L., Lengele, B., Morelon, E., Testelin, S., Michallet, M., D'Hauthuille, C. and Dubernard, J. (2006) First human face allograft: early report, *The Lancet*, 368: 203–9.

Dickenson, D. and Widdershoven, G. (2001) Ethical issues in limb transplants, *Bioethics*, 15(2): 110–24.

Dodd-McCue, D., Cowherd, R., Iveson, A. and Myer, K. (2006) Family responses to donor designation in donation cases: a longitudinal study, *Progress in Transplantation*, 16(2): 150–4.

Haire, M.C. and Hinchliff, J.P. (1996) Donation of heart valve tissue: seeking consent and meeting the needs of donor families, *Medical Journal of Australia*, 164: 28–31.

Kluge, E. H. (1997) Decisions about organ donation should rest with potential donors, not next of kin, *Canadian Medical Association*, 157(2): 160–1.

Lock, M. (2002) *Twice Dead: Organ Transplants and the Reinvention of Death.* Berkeley, CA: University of California Press.

Matesanz, R. and Miranda, B. (2002) A decade of continuous improvement in cadaveric organ donation: the Spanish model, *Journal of Nephrology*, 15: 22–8.

Niklason, L.E. and Langer, R. (2001) Prospects for organ and tissue replacement, *American Medical Association*, 285(5): 573–6.

Ramsay, S. (2001) 105,000 body parts retained in UK, census says, *The Lancet*, 357–65.

Redfern, M. (2001) *The Royal Liverpool Children's Inquiry Report*. London: The Stationery Office.

Retained Organs Commission (2002a) *External Review of Birmingham Children's Hospital NHS Trust: Report on Organ Retention*. London: DoH.

Retained Organs Commission (2002b) *Investigation into Organ Retention at Central Manchester and Manchester Children's University Hospitals*. London: DoH.

Retained Organs Commission (2002c) Proposals for identifying and meeting families support needs. Annex 1. Outline tender specification document: identifying and meeting the support needs of families affected by organ retention. Ninth meeting on the 30 May. (ROC 09/5).M. (2001) *The Royal Liverpool Children's Inquiry Report*. London: The Stationery Office.

Richardson, R. (2001) *Death, Dissection and the Destitute*, 2nd edn. Chicago: Chicago University Press.

Rumsey, N. (2004) Psychological aspects of face transplantation: read the small print carefully, *The American Journal of Bioethics*, 4(3): 22–5.

Scheper-Hughes, N. (2000) The global traffic in organs, *Current Anthropology*, 41(2): 191–224.

Spurgeon, B. (2005) Surgeons pleased with patient's progress after face transplant, *British Medical Journal*, 331: 1359.

Sque, M., Long, T. and Payne, S. (2004) *From Understanding to Implementation: Meeting the Needs of Families and Individuals Affected by Post Mortem Organ Retention. Final Report of a Study Commissioned by the Department of Health with the Retained Organs Commission*. University of Southampton, Southampton: UK.

Sque, M., Long, T. and Payne S. (2005) Organ donation: key factors influencing families' decision-making, *Transplantation Proceedings*, 37(2): 543–6.

Sque, M., Long, T., Payne, S. and Allardyce, D. (2006) *Exploring the End of Life Decision-making and Hospital Experiences of Families Who Did Not Donate Organs for Transplant Operations. Final Research Report for UK Transplant*. University of Southampton, Southampton: UK.

Tsai, R.J., Li, L.M. and Chen, J.K. (2000) Reconstruction of damaged corneas by transplantation of autologous limbal epithelial cells, *New England Journal of Medicine*, 343: 86–93.

UK Transplant (2005) *Annual Report 2004–2005*. http://www.uktransplant.org.uk/ukt/about_us/annual_report/annual_report.jsp (accessed 29 January 2006).

Youngner, S.J., Anderson, M.W. and Schapiro, R. (eds) (2004) *Transplanting Human Tissue: Ethics, Policy and Practice*. Oxford: Oxford University Press.

Appendix 1
Issues raised by the Human Tissue Act with regard to living donation

Patricia M. Franklin and Alison K. Crombie

Most European countries have laws permitting the use of living donor organs, and are therefore fundamentally supportive of the practice of live donation.

Legislation in the UK has until recently been perhaps the most prescriptive in Europe, partly because it was introduced to prohibit commercial dealings in human organs. As a direct consequence, living donor transplants in the UK are at present regulated by the Human Organ Transplants Act 1989. The Act goes considerably further than simply barring payment for organs for transplantation, it states that a person commits an offence if he or she removes an organ or transplants an organ from a living donor unless the recipient is genetically related to the donor. The Act defines very precisely what a genetically related donor means.

A person is genetically related to his or her natural parents and children; his or her brothers and sisters of the whole or half blood; the brothers and sisters of the whole or half blood of either of his or her natural parents; and the natural children of the brothers and sisters of the whole or half blood of either of his or her natural parents.

The Act does not, however, recognize grandparents or more distant relatives as genetically related. At the time of the Bill the Under Secretary announced that the Bill had been drafted to permit organ transplants between close relatives because there are clinical advantages, they are more likely to be compatible in a medical sense, and the motives of a donor, who is a relative, are more likely to be altruistic.

The Act also stated that before any related-donor transplant could take place, specified genetic testing of donor and recipient must prove the claimed genetic relationship. The Act did allow unrelated living donor transplants to be performed, but only after very considerable scrutiny. The Act established a Committee, the Unrelated Live Transplants Regulatory Authority (ULTRA), with power to authorize transplants between non-genetically related donors subject to certain conditions being met. An application to ULTRA had to contain full details of the donor, full details of the recipient (each report being written by a different clinician) and a report from an independent third clinician who was satisfied that the donor had 'understandable' and 'acceptable' motives for wishing to donate the organ, and in addition had not been coerced, bribed or induced to act as a donor for any unacceptable motives.

It has been suggested that the government, in their desire to stop all unacceptable living donor transplants, may have produced legislation that was 'Unnecessarily intrusive and difficult when clinicians try to arrange perfectly acceptable transplants' (Rudge 1996: 18). Yet the intention of the Bill was not to discourage emotionally-related donors. The Under Secretary, at the time, stated that he wished to make it plain that voluntary donation from genetically unrelated individuals was not being discouraged if their relative, spouse or friend was suffering from renal failure. The aim was to restrict donation to those that have a strong commitment through a close relationship.

In fact, as the Eurotold report (Donnelly and Price 1997) highlighted, it was somewhat anomalous that in Britain genetically unrelated donors, irrespective of their relationship with the recipient, were subject to greater mandatory screening and protection than related donors; yet related donors also have family influences bearing on the decision-making process. Further, there appeared to be an implicit assumption made that genetically-related persons were always outside the influence of commercial interests. In Britain, because commercialism is generally considered an evil to be avoided, spouses fall outside the definition of 'genetically related' (Donnelly and Price 1997). Further studies also highlighted this anomaly and suggested the need for all donors whether related or not related to have access to an independent donor advocate. Furthermore, this legislation did not allow for wider recruitment of unrelated donations such as paired-pooled donation and altruistic donation, which have been successfully undertaken in other countries. Therefore new legislation, the Human Tissue Act (2004), implemented in September 2006, replaced the Human Organs Transplant Act 1989.

The Human Tissue Act

The Human Tissue Authority (HTA) will regulate all living donor transplants. The role of the Independent Assessor (IA) will be key to the process of assessment of all live donations and the IA must be trained and accredited by the HTA.

The new legal framework will include all the previous related and unrelated relationships cited in 1989 but will also include those previously excluded by law, 'children', adults lacking capacity, paired-pooled donors and altruistic non-directed donors.

Paired-pooled donation

This group includes incompatible donor and recipient pairs who will be matched to other incompatible pairs either within the local unit or elsewhere in the UK. The potential donors will be assessed per national guidelines/local unit protocols and names submitted to the national register (UK Transplant for matching). Approval for this process will be through the HTA and simultaneous operations will be planned, maintaining anonymity for all parties.

Such paired-pooled donations have been reported from American and Scandinavian units and others and have proved to be successful in increasing the number of organs available, but strict ethical and practical considerations must apply.

Altruistic non-directed donation

The altruistic non-directed donors are donors who have no genetic or emotional relationship with the potential recipient. These are individuals who express a wish to help a stranger. These donors will also be assessed as per national/unit protocol and their name submitted to the national register (UK Transplant). The organ will be allocated to the recipient in line with approved allocation principles and after HTA approval the operation will be planned, maintaining anonymity for both parties.

The new Human Tissue Act mandates that all live donations are subject to assessment by an IA. IAs are trained professionals who act as a representative of the HTA and as an advocate for the donor. The advocate is required to ensure that the donor understands the nature of the medical procedure and the risks of the procedure, and consents to the removal of the organ in question. Furthermore, that the donor's consent has not been obtained by coercion or any other inducement, that there is no evidence of an offer or reward. In addition the donor must understand that they are entitled to withdraw their consent at any time, that the donor and recipient relationship is as stated and that there are no difficulties in communicating with the donor and recipient. If these exist the IA must clarify how these have been overcome.

To fulfil these legal requirements the responsibilities of the IA include an interview with the donor and recipient separately and together and the preparation of a report to show that all legal requirements have been met. The IA must be an NHS medical consultant or someone with an equivalent registered professional status and currently registered with a professional body. They must not be active in human organ transplantation and have no direct involvement with the transplant programme or any vested interest in transplantation. They must have completed the designated training and be accredited with the HTA.

The issues pertaining to all live donors in future having recourse to an IA have been welcomed by the transplant community and others as it has long been argued that related donation can also be subject to the same pressures and coercion as unrelated donation. As Price (1996) suggests it can provide an additional safeguard for all donors.

Summary

In summary, as Machado (1998) has asserted, it is clear that these regulations serve a variety of interests, responding to social and medical requirements, but they are also expressions of the significant weight and extent of legal control applied to private areas of human existence. Legislation not only regulates and legitimizes practices that make use of the body and body parts in clinical medicine and research, but also engenders legally sanctioned definitions of individual rights. Moreover, the regulation of live donation has implications far beyond the medical sphere in redefining the boundaries between individual rights, family rights and state rights in dealing with bodies and body parts.

References

Donnelly, P. and Price, D. (1997) *Questioning Attitudes to Living Donor Transplantation: European Multicentre Study Transplantation of Organs from Living Donors – ethical and legal dimensions*. Leicester: EUROTOLD Project Management Group.

Machado, N. (1998) *Using the Bodies of the Dead: Legal, Ethical and Organisational Dimensions of Organ Transplantation*. Dartmouth: Asgate.

Price, D.P.T. (1996) The voluntarism and informedness of living donors, in D.P.T. Price and H. Akveld (eds) *Living Organ Donation in the Nineties: European Medico-Legal Perspectives*. Leicester: European Commission.

Rudge, C. (1996) Policy issues relating to living donation in the United Kingdom, in D.P.T Price and H. Akveld (eds) *Living Organ Donation in the Nineties: European Medico-Legal Perspectives*. Leicester: European Commission.

Index